Asthma: Targeted Biological Therapies

Girolamo Pelaia · Alessandro Vatrella
Rosario Maselli

Asthma: Targeted Biological Therapies

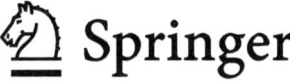 Springer

Girolamo Pelaia
University "Magna Graecia"
Catanzaro
Italy

Rosario Maselli
University "Magna Graecia"
Catanzaro
Italy

Alessandro Vatrella
University of Salerno
Salerno
Italy

ISBN 978-3-319-46005-5   ISBN 978-3-319-46007-9   (eBook)
DOI 10.1007/978-3-319-46007-9

Library of Congress Control Number: 2016958300

Printed on acid-free paper

This Springer imprint is published by Springer Nature
The registered company is Springer International Publishing AG Switzerland
The registered company address is Gewerbestrasse 11, 6330 Cham, Switzerland

Contents

1   **Introduction**.   1
    References.   3

2   **Inflammatory Cellular Patterns in Asthma**   5
    Eosinophilic Asthma.   5
    Neutrophilic Asthma.   8
    Mixed Granulocytic (Eosinophilic/Neutrophilic) Airway
    Inflammation.   10
    Paucigranulocytic Asthma   11
    Concluding Remarks.   11
    References.   12

3   **Airway Remodelling in Asthma**.   17
    Epithelial Changes   17
    Subepithelial Thickening   19
    Airway Smooth Muscle Remodelling.   20
    Increased Bronchial Vasculature.   21
    Concluding Remarks.   22
    References.   22

4   **Anti-IgE Therapy**   27
    Role of IgE in Allergic Asthma   27
    Omalizumab: Mechanism of Action and Pharmacokinetics.   31
    Therapeutic Use of Omalizumab as Add-On Treatment for Asthma   33
    Safety and Tolerability Profile of Omalizumab   39
    Cost-Effectiveness of Omalizumab Treatment for Severe Asthma   40
    Future Perspectives of Anti-IgE Therapy   41
    Concluding Remarks.   42
    References.   43

5   **IL-5-Targeted Antibodies**.   51
    Role of IL-5 in Eosinophilic Asthma   51
    Mepolizumab   53
    Reslizumab   56
    Benralizumab   59
    Concluding Remarks.   62
    References.   63

6   Anti-IL-4/IL-13 Biologics   67
   Role of IL-4 and IL-13 in Asthma Pathobiology   67
   IL-4-/IL-13-Targeted Therapies   69
      Pascolizumab   69
      Pitrakinra.   72
      Dupilumab.   72
      Anti-IL-4/IL-13 Bispecific Antibodies.   75
      Lebrikizumab   75
      Tralokinumab   77
      GSK679586.   78
   Concluding Remarks.   79
   References.   79

7   Anti-TNF-α Therapies   83
   References.   86

8   Biologic Treatments Targeted to Innate Cytokines   89
   Anti-IL-25 Monoclonal Antibodies   89
   Anti-IL-33 Therapies   89
   Anti-TSLP Treatments   90
   References.   90

9   Other Biologic Drugs   93
   Anti-IL-9 Monoclonal Antibodies   93
   Anti-GM-CSF Drugs   94
   Anti-IL-17 and Anti-IL-23 Therapies.   94
   References.   95

10 Conclusions and Future Perspectives   97
   References.   98

Asthma is a chronic respiratory disease, clinically manifesting as wheezing, shortness of breath and chest tightness, which is featured by bronchial obstruction mainly due to inflammatory and structural changes leading to airway hyperresponsiveness and acute bronchoconstriction [1, 2]. This widespread airway disorder affects over 300 million asthmatic people worldwide, which will probably become more than 400 million by 2020 [3, 4]. Rather than a single disease entity, asthma is currently believed to be a heterogeneous complex of multiple clinical and pathobiologic phenotypes, characterized by different responses to pharmacological therapies [5, 6]. The majority of asthmatic patients can achieve a good control of their symptoms using standard treatments including inhaled corticosteroids and bronchodilators such as β_2-adrenergic agonists, as well as oral leukotriene inhibitors [7, 8].

However, despite an optimized inhaled therapy, a minority of subjects with severe disease are not adequately controlled and experience frequent exacerbations. In addition, asthma severity in these difficult-to-treat patients is often further worsened by the coexistence of one or more comorbidities, including chronic rhinitis and sinusitis, gastro-oesophageal reflux, obesity, obstructive sleep apnoea (OSA) and even chronic obstructive pulmonary disease (COPD) [9]. Although when considering the overall population of asthmatic subjects, patients suffering from severe disease constitute a relatively small percentage, ranging from 5 to 10 %; however, they consume a huge share of economic resources, amounting to about 50 % of the global asthma budget (Fig. 1.1) [10–12]. This very high cost of severe asthma is caused by the frequent fruition of healthcare services such as unscheduled consultations and emergency visits, as well as additional consumption of drugs and hospitalizations for recurrent exacerbations. Furthermore, severe asthma is associated with significant losses of school- and workdays, and asthmatic subjects with uncontrolled disease often experience also anxiety and depression [13]. Therefore, patients expressing asthma phenotypes refractory to conventional treatments are characterized by the most urgent unmet medical needs, which thus require a close attention to the assessment, monitoring and therapeutic management of their disease.

The above considerations imply that though in many asthmatic patients standard treatments, and especially corticosteroids, are very effective because of their wide capability of interfering with several pro-inflammatory networks involved in asthma pathobiology, however various degrees of corticosteroid resistance can occur in severe asthma [14]. Indeed, corticosteroid insensitivity is one of the main concepts emphasized in the recent document focusing on severe asthma, jointly published by

© Springer International Publishing Switzerland 2017
G. Pelaia et al., *Asthma: Targeted Biological Therapies*,
DOI 10.1007/978-3-319-46007-9_1

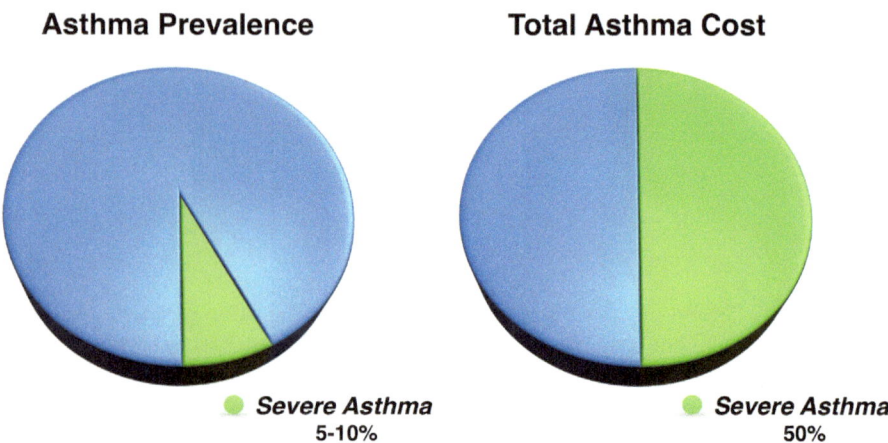

Asthma Prevalence   **Total Asthma Cost**

● *Severe Asthma*   ● *Severe Asthma*
5-10%   50%

Fig. 1.1 High cost of severe asthma

the European Respiratory Society (ERS) and the American Thoracic Society (ATS) [15]. Therefore, although in many asthmatic patients corticosteroids are very efficacious, they cannot be regarded as a 'one-size-fits-all' treatment. Hence, particularly in severe asthma, an accurate phenotypic characterization should be pursued, in order to pinpoint the relevant cellular and molecular targets involved in disease pathobiology [16]. Through such a personalized strategy, it would be possible to tailor individual therapies aimed to achieve an adequate and persistent control of symptoms, as well as to decrease the risk of future exacerbations and to slow down the progression of lung function decline [17]. Within this context, the present and future cornerstone of patient-centred treatment of severe asthma is based on the use of biologic drugs [18–21]. Biological therapies usually include monoclonal antibodies, soluble receptors and genetically altered cytokines. The first biologic compound approved for treatment of uncontrolled asthma was omalizumab, a humanized monoclonal antibody directed against human immunoglobulin E (IgE), which plays a pivotal pathogenic role in allergic asthma [22–25]. The anti-IgE therapy with omalizumab is recommended by Global Initiative for Asthma (GINA) guidelines at step 5, referring to severe asthma [26]. GINA step 5 now also includes mepolizumab [26], a humanized monoclonal antibody targeted towards interleukin-5 (IL-5), the main cytokine responsible for maturation, activation and survival of eosinophils. Other biologics are in advanced stages of clinical investigation, and they will probably be introduced in clinical practice within the next few years. These new antiasthma biologic drugs mainly target Th2 cell-derived cytokines (IL-4, IL-5, IL-13) or their receptors [27]. Because biologic treatments for asthma point to specific molecular and cellular targets, eligible patients should be identified through a search for reliable and easily assessable biomarkers. Among these, the most commonly measured in asthmatic patients are serum IgE, sputum and especially blood eosinophils, fractional exhaled nitric oxide (FeNO) and periostin, a matricellular protein produced by both inflammatory and airway structural cells upon stimulation by Th2 cytokines

[28, 29]. In addition to the biomarkers routinely detectable in clinical practice, for research purposes, a further valuable contribution to a better phenotypic characterization of asthmatic patients can undoubtedly be provided by more sophisticated experimental approaches based on the so-called 'omics' technologies such as genomics, metabolomics and proteomics [30, 31]. In particular, because proteins, and not genes, are responsible for the overall complexity of an organism, proteomics is especially useful to characterize the different phenotypic patterns of asthma [32, 33]. Therefore, this molecular approach can significantly help to delineate the pathogenetic substrates of clinical phenotypes, thus figuring out the so-called endotypes, defined as disease subgroups featured by specific pathophysiologic connotates. Such a conceptual evolution from phenotypes to endotypes, linking the clinical presentations of asthma to their underlying pathobiology, is crucial for the current efforts aimed at identifying the molecular targets towards which biological therapies are pointed [34, 35]. Indeed, identification of genomic and/or proteomic biomarkers plays a pivotal role for the discovery of suitable therapeutic targets. On the other hand, a careful individual search for already known biomarkers is essential for the success of 'precision' medicines like biologic drugs. Through this personalized approach, it is thereby possible to find patient groups with specific phenotypes/endotypes of asthma, especially suffering from severe and uncontrolled disease, who are potentially responsive to targeted biologic treatments able to markedly alleviate their symptoms, as well as to decrease the frequency and severity of their exacerbations.

On the basis of the above-mentioned considerations, the aim of this concise book is to outline and discuss, after recalling recent knowledge about airway inflammation and remodelling, the currently used and newly developed biological therapies for severe asthma.

References

1. Holgate ST, Wenzel S, Postma DS, et al. Asthma. Nat Rev Dis Primers. 2015;1:15025.
2. Pelaia G, Vatrella A, Busceti MT, et al. Cellular mechanisms underlying eosinophilic and neutrophilic airway inflammation in asthma. Mediators Inflamm. 2015:879783. doi: 10.1155/2015/879783. Epub 2015 Mar 23.
3. Masoli M, Fabian D, Holt S, et al. The global burden of asthma: executive summary of the GINA dissemination committee report. Allergy. 2010;59:469–78.
4. Chanez P, Humbert M. Asthma: still a promising future? Eur Respir Rev. 2014;23:405–7.
5. Ray A, Oriss TB, Wenzel SE. Emerging molecular phenotypes of asthma. Am J Physiol Lung Cell Mol Physiol. 2015;308:L130–40.
6. Gauthier M, Ray A, Wenzel SE. Evolving concepts of asthma. Am J Respir Crit Care Med. 2015;192:660–8.
7. Bateman ED, Boushey HA, Bousquet J, et al. Can guideline-defined asthma control be achieved? The Gaining Optimal Asthma ControL (GOAL) study. Am J Respir Crit Care Med. 2004;170:836–44.
8. Fanta CH. Drug therapy: asthma. N Engl J Med. 2009;360:1002–14.
9. Boulet LP. Influence of comorbid conditions on asthma. Eur Respir J. 2009;33:897–906.
10. Serra-Batlles J, Plaza V, Morejon E, et al. Costs of asthma according to the degree of severity. Eur Respir J. 1998;12:1322–6.

11. Antonicelli L, Bucca C, Neri M, et al. Asthma severity and medical resource utilisation. Eur Respir J. 2004;23:723–9.
12. Accordini S, Corsico AG, Braggion M, et al. The cost of persistent asthma in Europe: an international population-based study in adults. Int Arch Allergy Immunol. 2013;160:93–101.
13. Heaney LG, Conway E, Kelly C, et al. Predictors of therapy resistant asthma: outcome of a systematic evaluation protocol. Thorax. 2003;58:561–6.
14. Barnes PJ. Corticosteroid resistance in patients with asthma and chronic obstructive pulmonary disease. J Allergy Clin Immunol. 2013;131:636–43.
15. Chung KF, Wenzel SE, Brozek JL, et al. International ERS/ATS guidelines on definition, evaluation and treatment of severe asthma. Eur Respir J. 2014;43:343–73.
16. Ray A, Raundhal M, Oriss TB, et al. Current concepts of severe asthma. J Clin Invest. 2016;126:2394–403.
17. Reddel HK, Bateman ED, Becker A, et al. A summary of the new GINA strategy: a roadmap to asthma control. Eur Respir J. 2015;46:622–39.
18. Pelaia G, Vatrella A, Maselli R. The potential of biologics for the treatment of asthma. Nat Rev Drug Discov. 2012;11:958–72.
19. Fajt ML, Wenzel SE. Biologic therapy in asthma: entering the new age of personalized medicine. J Asthma. 2014;51:669–76.
20. Darveaux J, Busse WW. Biologics in asthma – the next step toward personalized medicine. J Allergy Clin Immunol Pract. 2015;3:152–60.
21. Fajt ML, Wenzel SE. Asthma phenotypes and the use of biologic medications in asthma and allergic disease: the next step toward personalized care. J Allergy Clin Immunol. 2015;135:299–310.
22. Gould HJ, Sutton BJ. IgE in allergy and asthma today. Nat Rev Immunol. 2008;8:205–17.
23. Dullaers M, De Bruyne R, Ramadani F, et al. The who, where and when of IgE in allergic airway disease. J Allergy Clin Immunol. 2012;129:635–45.
24. Humbert M, Busse W, Hanania NA, et al. Omalizumab in asthma: an update on recent developments. J Allergy Clin Immunol Pract. 2014;2:525–36.
25. Pelaia G, Vatrella A, Busceti MT, et al. Anti-IgE therapy with omalizumab for severe asthma: current concepts and potential developments. Curr Drug Targets. 2015;16:171–8.
26. Global strategy for asthma management and prevention. Global Initiative for Asthma (GINA). 2016. Available from: http://www.ginasthma.org/.
27. Gallelli L, Busceti MT, Vatrella A, et al. Update on anticytokine treatment for asthma. Biomed Res Int. 2013:104315. doi: 10.1155/2013/104315. Epub 2013 Jun 18.
28. Szefler SJ, Wenzel S, Brown R, et al. Asthma outcomes: biomarkers. J Allergy Clin Immunol. 2012;129:S9–23.
29. Li W, Gao P, Zhi Y, et al. Periostin: its role in asthma and its potential as a diagnostic or therapeutic target. Respir Res. 2015;16:57.
30. Rossi R, De Palma A, Benazzi L, et al. Biomarker discovery in asthma and COPD by proteomic approaches. Proteomics Clin Appl. 2014;8:901–15.
31. Terracciano R, Pelaia G, Preianò M, et al. Asthma and COPD proteomics: current approaches and future directions. Proteomics Clin Appl. 2015;9:203–20.
32. Houtman R, van den Worm E. Asthma, the ugly duckling of lung disease proteomics? J Chromatogr B. 2005;815:285–94.
33. Bowler RP, Ellison MC, Reisdorph N. Proteomics in pulmonary medicine. Chest. 2006;130:567–74.
34. Anderson GP. Endotyping asthma: new insights into key pathogenetic mechanisms in a complex, heterogeneous disease. Lancet. 2008;372:1107–19.
35. Xie M, Wenzel SE. A global perspective in asthma: from phenotype to endotype. Chin Med J. 2013;126:166–74.

Airway inflammation, sustained by a multitude of pro-inflammatory mediators such as cytokines and chemokines produced by both immune-inflammatory and airway structural cells, is a hallmark of asthma [1, 2]. Several inflammatory phenotypes of asthma have been characterized, which include eosinophilic, neutrophilic, mixed and paucigranulocytic patterns [3, 4]. Eosinophils are the inflammatory cells most frequently infiltrating the airways of asthmatic patients; indeed, their maturation, activation, survival and recruitment within the bronchial wall and airway lumen are crucially implicated in the development of both allergic and non-allergic asthma [5, 6]. Eosinophilic asthma originates from the activation of immunopathologic and pro-inflammatory pathways, mainly coordinated by T-helper 2 (Th2) lymphocytes, which release interleukin-5, interleukin-4 and interleukin-13 (IL-5, IL-4 and IL-13) (Fig. 2.1). In addition to being driven by adaptive immune responses, airway eosinophilia can also arise from innate immune mechanisms, which are mediated by intercellular communications involving dendritic cells, bronchial epithelial cells and innate lymphoid cells [7, 8]. Whilst bronchial eosinophilic infiltration is mostly responsible for mild-to-moderate asthma, more severe disease is often characterized by mixed patterns of inflammation including both eosinophils and neutrophils, with the latter which can represent the predominant inflammatory cells detectable in the induced sputum obtained from patients experiencing uncontrolled asthmatic symptoms and exacerbations. Neutrophilic airway inflammation, associated with severe asthma, is triggered by Th1 and especially Th17 lymphocytes (Fig. 2.1) [9, 10]. Within this pathobiologic context, a pivotal role is played by dendritic cells, which direct the commitment to the various Th lineages. In particular, polarization towards the different Th subsets is closely linked to the particular airway milieu consisting of specific co-stimulatory molecules and cytokines, which drive the various Th cell programmes [11].

Eosinophilic Asthma

Eosinophilic airway inflammation underlies the clinical phenotype of early-onset allergic asthma, as well as the development and progression of late-onset non-allergic asthma.

Allergic asthma is implemented by an immune-inflammatory response induced by Th2 cells. This so-called 'Th2-high' or 'type 2' sub-phenotype of asthma arises

© Springer International Publishing Switzerland 2017   5
G. Pelaia et al., *Asthma: Targeted Biological Therapies*,
DOI 10.1007/978-3-319-46007-9_2

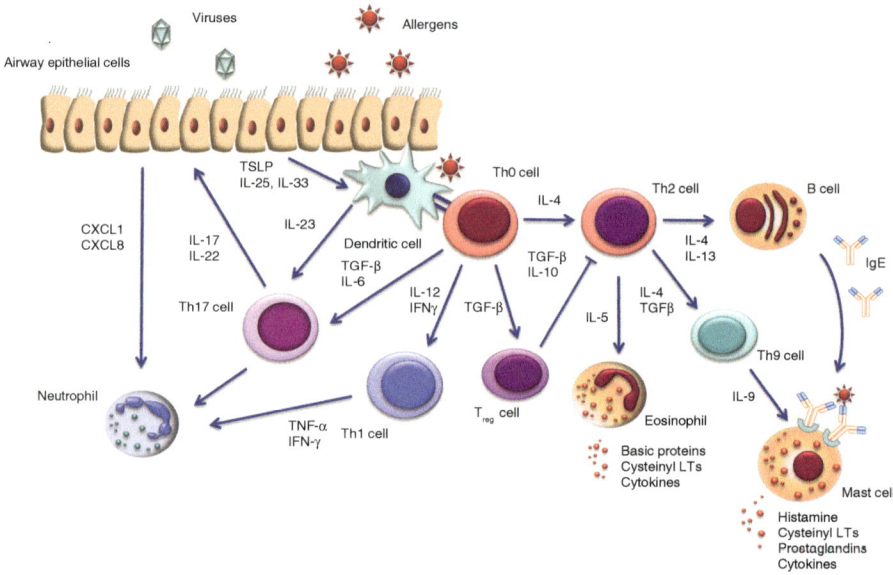

Fig. 2.1 Pathobiology of airway inflammation in asthma. Asthma originates from complex interactions between genetic factors and environmental agents such as aeroallergens and respiratory viruses. In particular, within the airway lumen, allergens can be captured by dendritic cells, which process antigenic molecules and present them to naïve (Th0) T-helper cells. The consequent activation of allergen-specific Th2 cells is responsible for the production of IL-4 and IL-13 that promote B-cell-operated synthesis of IgE antibodies; moreover, Th2 cells also release IL-5, which induces eosinophil maturation and survival. These events are noticeably favoured by a functional defect of IL-10/TGF-β producing T regulatory (Treg) cells that normally exert an immunosuppressive action on Th2 cell-mediated responses. In addition to Th2 cells, IL-9 releasing Th9 cells can also undergo activation, thus leading to the growth and recruitment of mast cells, which upon IgE-dependent degranulation release both preformed and newly synthesized mediators. Other important T lymphocytes contributing to asthma pathobiology are Th17 cells, producing IL17A and IL-17F which cause neutrophil recruitment and expansion. Furthermore, IL-12-dependent, IFN-γ-releasing Th1 cells can be activated, especially as a result of airway infections sustained by respiratory viruses. Abbreviations: *CXCL1* chemokine CXC motif ligand 1, *CXCL8* chemokine CXC motif ligand 8, *TNF-α* tumour necrosis factor-α, *TSLP* thymic stromal lymphopoietin (Modified from Ref. [4])

from complex interactions between the innate and adaptive branches of the immune system [12, 13]. Differentiation of Th2 lymphocytes depends on a mutual cooperation involving several promoting factors, including co-stimulatory molecules and cytokines expressed by dendritic cells and inflammatory cells. In particular, aeroallergens which trigger allergic asthma, including pollens, house-dust mite and animal dander, are frequently featured by proteolytic properties and also contain trace amounts of bacterial constituents such as lipopolysaccharide (LPS) [14]. Therefore, once penetrated into the airway epithelium, inhaled allergens can stimulate the Toll-like receptor (TLR) class of pattern recognition receptors implicated in innate immunity. TLR activation induces the epithelial synthesis of innate cytokines such as thymic stromal lymphopoietin (TSLP), IL-25 and IL-33, able to induce the development of Th2 adaptive responses (Fig. 2.1). IL-33 can also be produced by dendritic cells [15]. Furthermore, TLR stimulation also elicits the epithelial release of C-C chemokine ligands 2 (CCL2) and 20 (CCL20), which promote the recruitment and maturation of dendritic cells [12]. The latter extend their intraepithelial processes into the airway lumen, capture aeroallergens and process them inside the cytoplasm, thus generating allergenic peptide fragments. These are then loaded within the context of HLA molecules belonging to the class II of the major histocompatibility complex (MHC class II) expressed by dendritic cells, which migrate to T-cell areas of regional thoracic lymph nodes where antigen presentation to T lymphocytes takes place. Recognition of specific antigenic peptides by T-cell receptors triggers sensitization and the following adaptive immune response. Allergen-dependent activation of naïve T lymphocytes requires the interaction of their co-stimulatory molecules (CD28, ICOS, OX40) with the respective counter ligands expressed by dendritic cells (CD80/B7.1, CD86/B7.2, ICOS ligand, OX40 ligand) [16]. The type of antigen presentation-dependent commitment of T lymphocytes is crucially determined by the cytokine milieu. In particular, Th2 polarization needs a microenvironment characterized by high concentrations of IL-4 and low levels of IL-12. IL-4 is produced by mast cells and basophils, but not by dendritic cells [17]. GATA3 is the key transcription factor, expressed by Th2 lymphocytes, that drives the synthesis of Th2 cytokines. The latter include IL-4, IL-5, IL-9 and IL-13. These cytokines stimulate the maturation and recruitment of other immune cells involved in the allergic cascade, such as eosinophils and mast cells [18]. In particular, IL-4 and IL-13 act on B lymphocytes by driving immunoglobulin class switching towards the production of IgE (Fig. 2.1) [1, 2]. IL-9, secreted by a further subset of T lymphocytes (Th9) derived from Th2 cells, attracts mast cells and triggers their differentiation (Fig. 2.1) [19].

IL-5 plays a key role in inducing the differentiation and maturation of eosinophils in bone marrow, as well as their activation and survival [20]. Transendothelial migration of eosinophils to the airways of patients with allergic asthma is stimulated by IL-4 via induction of vascular cell adhesion molecule-1 (VCAM-1), which specifically interacts with its eosinophil counter ligand very late antigen-4 (VLA-4). In chronic allergic asthma, IgE-activated mast cells persistently secrete eosinophil recruiting cytokines (e.g. IL-3, IL-4, IL-5, GM-CSF), whose action is synergized by several chemokines such as eotaxin 1/eotaxin 2 (CCL11/CCL24) and regulated upon activation, normal T cell expressed and secreted (RANTES) [21, 22]. As a consequence, the prolonged eosinophil infiltration and degranulation result in a continuous release of cytotoxic products including major basic protein, eosinophil cationic protein, eosinophil-derived neurotoxin and eosinophil peroxidase, which significantly contribute to airway epithelial damage, mucus overproduction from goblet cells, bronchial hyperresponsiveness and impaired ciliary beating. Moreover, eosinophils secrete cysteinyl leukotrienes (LTC_4, LTD_4 and LTE_4), powerful pro-inflammatory mediators which induce bronchoconstriction, mucus hypersecretion and activation of eosinophils themselves [23–26]. In addition to producing many pro-inflammatory mediators, eosinophils contribute to allergic asthmatic inflammation also by acting as antigen-presenting cells [27], thereby exposing allergen peptides to T lymphocytes.

The late-onset variant of eosinophilic asthma, which occurs at adulthood, is often non-allergic. Indeed, this particular disease phenotype frequently develops in the absence of allergen-dependent activation of Th2 lymphocytes. Current evidence suggests that a central function in coordinating eosinophilic non-allergic asthma is exerted by the group 2 innate lymphoid cells (ILC2s), whose differentiation depends on the expression of the transcription factor RORα [5, 6, 8]. Following stimulation elicited by TSLP, IL-25 and IL-33, ILC2s release Th2-type cytokines including large quantities of IL-5 and IL-13, but much less IL-4 [28–30]. Production of Th2-type cytokines by these cells is also stimulated by prostaglandin D_2 (PGD_2) via activation of its chemoattractant receptor-homologous molecule expressed on Th2 cell (CRTH2) receptor, which is expressed by ILC2s [31]. High levels of ILC2s have been found in eosinophilic nasal polyps, as well as in peripheral blood and induced sputum of asthmatic patients with persistent airway eosinophilia [32–34]. Furthermore, in murine experimental models of asthma induced by either influenza A virus or the fungus *Alternaria alternata*, characterized by airway eosinophilia, it was shown that ILC2s were required and sufficient to cause eosinophil recruitment and bronchial hyperresponsiveness, independently of Th2 cells [35, 36].

Therefore, two different and nonmutually exclusive pro-inflammatory pathways activated by either allergen-specific Th2 lymphocytes or allergen-independent innate ILC2s, both leading to IL-5 production, are responsible for eosinophilic airway inflammation in asthma. IL-5, together with other survival factors such as IL-3, GM-CSF, IL-25, IL-33 and TSLP, delays eosinophil apoptosis [22]. Eosinophil apoptosis is induced by lipoxin A4, an arachidonic acid metabolite that inhibits IL-5 production and whose levels have been found to be decreased in the exhaled breath condensate of patients with asthma undergoing disease exacerbations [22, 37]. From a therapeutic point of view, corticosteroids are powerful inducers of eosinophil apoptosis [38], and this pro-apoptotic action represents one of the most effective antiasthma mechanisms of these drugs. Inhaled corticosteroids, which are the cornerstone of asthma treatment, cause eosinophil apoptosis by suppressing the synthesis of important eosinophil survival factors such as IL-3, IL-5 and GM-CSF [39, 40]. However, some patients with severe, uncontrolled eosinophilic asthma can exhibit various degrees of corticosteroid resistance. In these cases, an alternative anti-eosinophil pharmacological approach might be based on the use of biologic drugs directed against IL-5 or its receptor [41–43]. Therefore, eosinophils are strategic cellular targets of paramount importance for the treatment of airway inflammation in both allergic and non-allergic asthma.

Neutrophilic Asthma

Whilst Th2 lymphocytes are mainly involved in the development of eosinophilic allergic asthma, other Th cell subsets induce airway neutrophilic inflammation, often associated with the most severe asthmatic phenotypes [44]. In particular, a specific lineage of CD4$^+$ effector T lymphocytes, expressing IL-17 and thus named Th17, appears to play a key role in airway neutrophilia (Fig. 2.1) [9, 45]. Indeed, in lung tissue sections from asthmatic patients, there is an overexpression of IL-17A and IL-17F, whose levels correlate with asthma severity, especially in subjects with neutrophilic, steroid-resistant disease [46]. Differentiation of Th17 lymphocytes requires a composite mixture of cytokines and co-stimulatory signals, operating in the presence of high antigen concentrations which induce CD40 ligand (CD40L) expression on naïve T cells [47]. The interaction of CD40L with CD40 molecules exposed by dendritic cells also expressing CD86 will lead to Th17 polarization only within a cytokine milieu including IL-1β, IL-6 and TGF-β [11, 48]. These cytokines are responsible for T-cell up-regulation of the master transcription factor RORγt, which is specific for Th17 commitment, as well as for the overexpression of IL-23 receptor [48, 49]. IL-23 is indeed crucial for maintaining Th17 cells in a functionally active state [50]. Allergens and other environmental stimuli such as cigarette smoke and diesel exhaust particles have been shown to trigger Th17-mediated airway inflammation in asthmatic subjects [11]. Indeed, cigarette smoking is often associated with bronchial neutrophilia, more severe asthma and corticosteroid insensitivity [51, 52]. In addition to cigarette smoke and airborne pollutants, other environmental agents such as microbes and microbial particles have also been implicated in the development of severe asthma [11]. In this regard, a relevant pathogenic role in Th17 cell-associated severe asthma could be played by the nucleotide-binding oligomerization domain-like receptor family, pyrin domain containing 3 activation (NLRP3) inflammasome, an intracellular multiprotein complex that facilitates the autoactivation of the pro-inflammatory cysteine protease caspase-1 [53, 54]. NRLP3 is activated by serum amyloid A (SAA) protein, which is produced upon exposure of airway epithelial cells to microbes and is detectable at high concentrations in both serum and induced sputum of asthmatic patients [55]. Asthmatic subjects are very susceptible to airway microbial burden, and both viral and bacterial components act as pathogen-associated molecular patterns (PAMPs), which are recognized by Toll-like receptors (TLRs) [53, 54]. The latter activate the transcription factor nuclear factor-kB (NF-kB), which induces the expression of pro-IL-1β and pro-IL-18 cytokines. The subsequent assembly of the NLRP3 inflammasome leads to activation of caspase-1, which cleaves pro-IL-1β and pro-IL-18, thus converting them in their mature forms [53, 54]; through this mechanism, active IL-1β can thus contribute to promote Th17 cell-dependent inflammation. Such a cascade of intracellular events, leading to NLRP3 activation, can also be triggered by danger-associated molecular patterns (DAMPs) [56], alarm signals that, for example, originate as a consequence of airway epithelial damage induced by oxidative stress associated with cigarette smoking and airborne pollutants. NLRP3 and caspase-1 protein have been found to be expressed in sputum neutrophils and macrophages from subjects with neutrophilic asthma [57]. Activation of the NLRP3 inflammasome can also occur in obesity-associated airway hyperresponsiveness [58].

Besides Th17 lymphocytes, other cellular sources of IL-17 include γδ T cells, cytotoxic T cells, invariant NK T cells, NK cells and group 3 innate lymphoid cells

(ILC3s) [8, 59]; the latter, which require RORγt and GATA3 transcription factors for their development, can be detected in the bronchoalveolar lavage (BAL) fluid from patients with severe asthma [8, 60]. Whatever are their cellular sources (e.g. Th17 cells and ILC3s), once released IL-17A and/or IL-17F stimulate airway structural cells, including bronchial epithelial cells and subepithelial fibroblasts, to secrete powerful neutrophil chemoattractants such as IL-8 (CXCL8) and CXCL1/ GRO-α [61–63]. These pro-inflammatory effects are mediated by stimulation of a receptor complex consisting of IL-17 receptor A (IL-17RA) and IL-17 receptor C (IL-17RC) subunits, coupled to a signalling network leading to NF-kB activation [64]. Th17 cell-associated neutrophilic asthma is often characterized by severe clinical forms, which are very difficult to manage because of a frequent steroid resistance. Indeed, differently from their pro-apoptotic action exerted on eosinophils, corticosteroids inhibit neutrophil apoptosis, thereby prolonging the survival of these inflammatory cells [65]. Thus, novel anti-neutrophil therapies are extremely needed for treatment of severe neutrophilic asthma.

Before the discovery of Th17 lymphocytes, Th1 cells, whose differentiation is driven by dendritic cells producing IL-12 and type 1 interferons and requires the expression of the specific transcription factor T-bet, were believed to be the main cellular coordinators of neutrophilic asthma [11, 66]. Indeed, Th1 cells and the Th1-derived cytokines interferon-γ (IFN-γ) and tumour necrosis factor-α (TNF-α) are increased in patients with severe asthma, and these observations suggested that Th1 cells could contribute to the development of airway neutrophilic inflammation (Fig. 2.1) [11, 67].

Mixed Granulocytic (Eosinophilic/Neutrophilic) Airway Inflammation

A concomitant activation of both Th2 and Th17 cells is associated with a mixed eosinophilic/neutrophilic inflammatory pattern, which often underlies the most severe asthma phenotypes. In this regard, Cosmi et al. identified in asthmatic patients the existence of circulating Th17/Th2 cell clones able to produce both IL-17A and IL-4 [68]. Within this conceptually new immunopathologic framework, Irvine et al. recently found in bronchoalveolar lavage (BAL) fluid from subjects with severe asthma, relatively high levels of dual-positive Th2/Th17 cells releasing large amounts of IL-4 and IL-17 [69]. Moreover, these authors detected in BAL lymphocytes a coexpression of both GATA3 and RORγt, namely, the transcription factors responsible for Th2 and Th17 cell differentiation, respectively [69]. Taken together, these findings corroborate previous results obtained in mice by Wang et al. who showed that Th2/Th17 cells induce a more severe form of experimental asthma [70]. Therefore, such novel findings require further studies aimed to better characterize these Th2/Th17 lymphocyte subpopulations and to more deeply elucidate the eventual additive or synergistic actions of Th2-/Th17-derived cytokines [71].

Paucigranulocytic Asthma

In addition to persistent airway eosinophilia and/or neutrophilia, on endobronchial biopsies obtained from subjects with severe asthma a further histopathological phenotype has been identified, which is defined as paucigranulocytic asthma [72, 73]. In particular, submucosal oedema and mucus hypersecretion can be detected in the airways of some asthmatic patients, in the absence of a demonstrable influx of eosinophils or neutrophils. The pathogenesis of this subtype of asthma is poorly understood. In these cases, inflammation could be caused by a pro-inflammatory activation of structural cellular elements such as bronchial epithelial cells and/or airway smooth muscle cells. However, during asthma exacerbations occurring in these patients, inflammation intensifies and can acquire granulocytic aspects [73].

Concluding Remarks

Airway inflammation, a key feature of asthma, is driven by complex cellular and molecular mechanisms leading to eosinophilic and/or neutrophilic bronchial infiltration, mainly dependent on Th2 and Th17 cell differentiation and activation, respectively (Fig. 2.1). Within this pathophysiologic context, a central role is played by dendritic cells, which direct the commitment of different Th cell lineages responsible for activation and recruitment into the airways of eosinophils and neutrophils [11]. Globally, these events occur in asthma as a consequence of the defective function of specific regulatory T lymphocytes (Treg cells) [74–76]. Several different Treg lymphocyte subsets have been identified, including naturally occurring CD4+CD25+ cells expressing the transcription factor FOXP3. Treg cells exert their immunomodulatory functions through direct and indirect mechanisms. In particular, Treg cells produce anti-inflammatory cytokines like IL-10 and TGF-β (Fig. 2.1), express inhibitory factors such as cytotoxic T lymphocyte antigen 4 (CTLA4) and also downregulate MHC class II proteins and CD80/CD86 co-stimulatory molecules expressed by antigen-presenting cells [77]. Because Treg cells directly or indirectly inhibit pro-inflammatory dendritic cells and promote the generation of tolerogenic dendritic cells, thus preventing the activation of effector Th1, Th2 and Th17 lymphocytes [76], the functional impairment of Treg-mediated immunomodulation makes asthmatic patients susceptible to the development of eosinophilic and neutrophilic bronchial inflammation. In particular, combined patterns of both neutrophilic and eosinophilic airway infiltrates may often coexist in severe asthma and in recurrent acute disease relapses that characterize the so-called exacerbation-prone asthmatic phenotype [78]. These exacerbations can be caused by allergens and especially by respiratory viruses, whose pathogenic effects within the airways of asthmatic subjects are favoured by a deficient epithelial synthesis of antiviral cytokines such as interferon-β (IFN-β) and interferon-λ (IFN-λ) [79, 80].

Therefore, it is undoubtable that a better knowledge of the intricate pathobiologic networks underlying the onset and progression of airway inflammation in asthma will pave the way for substantial improvements in the treatment of this widespread and sometimes severe disease. In particular, future research should focus on the development of prevention strategies and therapeutic options aimed to restore the impaired balance between immunosuppressive Treg lymphocytes and the various branches of asthma-inducing adaptive immunity, especially referring to Th2- and Th17-mediated responses. Such efforts should lead to widen and improve the currently available immunological and pharmacological approaches. In this regard, biological therapies could eventually provide the tools for personalized anti-asthma medications, capable of satisfying the individual needs of patients expressing distinct disease phenotypes.

References

1. Barnes PJ. The cytokine network in asthma and chronic obstructive pulmonary disease. J Clin Invest. 2008;118:3546–56.
2. Pawankar R, Hayashi M, Yamanishi S, et al. The paradigm of cytokine networks in allergic airway inflammation. Curr Opin Allergy Clin Immunol. 2015;15:41–8.
3. Wenzel SE. Complex phenotypes in asthma: current definitions. Pulm Pharmacol Ther. 2013;26:710–5.
4. Pelaia G, Vatrella A, Busceti MT, et al. Cellular mechanisms underlying eosinophilic and neutrophilic airway inflammation in asthma. Mediators Inflamm. 2015;2015:879783.
5. Lambrecht BN, Hammad H. The immunology of asthma. Nat Immunol. 2015;16:45–54.
6. Brusselle GG, Maes T, Bracke KR. Eosinophilic airway inflammation in nonallergic asthma. Nat Med. 2013;19:977–9.
7. Erle DJ, Sheppard D. The cell biology of asthma. J Cell Biol. 2014;205:621–31.
8. Yu S, Kim HY, Chang Ya J, et al. Innate lymphoid cells and asthma. J Allergy Clin Immunol. 2014;133:943–50.
9. Aujla SJ, Alcorn JF. T_H17 cells in asthma and inflammation. Biochim Biophys Acta. 2011;1810:1066–79.
10. Trejo Bittar HE, Yousem SA, Wenzel SE. Pathobiology of severe asthma. Annu Rev Pathol. 2015;10:511–45.
11. Vroman H, van den Blink B, Kool M. Mode of dendritic cell activation: the decisive hand in Th2/Th17 cell differentiation. Implications in asthma severity? Immunobiology. 2015;220:254–61.
12. Hammad H, Chieppa M, Perros F, et al. House dust mite allergen induces asthma via Toll-like receptor 4 triggering of airway structural cells. Nat Med. 2009;15:410–6.
13. Woodruff PG, Modrek B, Choy DF, et al. T-helper type 2-driven inflammation defines major sub-phenotypes of asthma. Am J Respir Crit Care Med. 2009;180:388–95.
14. Lloyd CM. Dust mites' dirty dealings in the lung. Nat Med. 2009;15:366–7.
15. Su Z, Lin J, Lu F, et al. Potential autocrine regulation of IL-33-ST2 signaling of dendritic cells in allergic inflammation. Mucosal Immunol. 2013;6:921–30.
16. Kallinich T, Beier KC, Wahn U, et al. T-cell co-stimulatory molecules: their role in allergic immune reactions. Eur Respir J. 2007;29:1246–55.
17. Kaiko GE, Horvat JC, Beagley KW, et al. Immunological decision-making: how does the immune system decide to mount a helper T-cell response? Immunology. 2008;123:326–38.
18. Larché M, Robinson DS, Kay AB. The role of T lymphocytes in the pathogenesis of asthma. J Allergy Clin Immunol. 2003;111:450–63.
19. Kaiko GE, Foster PS. New insights into the generation of Th2 immunity and potential therapeutic targets for the treatment of asthma. Curr Opin Allergy Clin Immunol. 2011;11:39–45.

20. Fulkerson PC, Rothenberg ME. Targeting eosinophils in allergy, inflammation and beyond. Nat Rev Drug Discov. 2013;12:117–29.
21. Park YM, Bochner BS. Eosinophil survival and apoptosis in health and disease. Allergy Asthma Immunol Res. 2010;2:87–101.
22. Felton JM, Lucas CD, Rossi AG, et al. Eosinophils in the lung – modulating apoptosis and efferocytosis in airway inflammation. Front Immunol. 2014;5:302.
23. Bandeira-Melo C, Bozza PT, Weller PF. The cellular biology of eosinophil eicosanoid formation and function. J Allergy Clin Immunol. 2002;109:393–400.
24. Peters-Golden M. Leukotrienes. N Engl J Med. 2007;357:1841–54.
25. Hallstrand TS, Henderson Jr WR. An update on the role of leukotrienes in asthma. Curr Opin Allergy Clin Immunol. 2010;10:60–6.
26. Hall S, Agrawal DK. Key mediators in the immunopathogenesis of allergic asthma. Int Immunopharmacol. 2014;23:316–29.
27. Jacobsen EA, Helmers RA, Lee JJ, et al. The expanding role(s) of eosinophils in health and disease. Blood. 2012;120:3882–90.
28. Walker JA, Barlow JL, McKenzie AN. Innate lymphoid cells: how did we miss them? Nat Rev Immunol. 2013;13:75–87.
29. McKenzie AN, Spits H, Eberl G. Innate lymphoid cells in inflammation and immunity. Immunity. 2014;41:366–74.
30. Karta MR, Broide DH, Doherty TA. Insights into group 2 innate lymphoid cells in human airway disease. Curr Allergy Asthma Rep. 2016;16:8.
31. Xue L, Salimi M, Panse I, et al. Prostaglandin D_2 activates group 2 innate lymphoid cells through chemoattractant receptor-homologous molecule expressed on T_H2 cells. J Allergy Clin Immunol. 2014;133:1184–94.
32. Mjosberg JM, Trifari S, Crellin NK, et al. Human IL-25- and IL-33-responsive type 2 innate lymphoid cells are defined by expression of CRTH2 and CD161. Nat Immunol. 2011;12:1055–62.
33. Bartemes KR, Kephart GM, Fox SJ, et al. Enhanced innate type 2 immune response in peripheral blood from patients with asthma. J Allergy Clin Immunol. 2014;134:671–8.
34. Smith SG, Chen R, Kjarsgaard M, et al. Increased numbers of activated group 2 innate lymphoid cells in the airways of patients with severe asthma and persistent airway eosinophilia. J Allergy Clin Immunol. 2016;137:75–86.
35. Chang YJ, Kim HY, Albacker LA, et al. Innate lymphoid cells mediate influenza-induced airway hyper-reactivity independently of adaptive immunity. Nat Immunol. 2011;12:631–8.
36. Bartemes KR, Iijima K, Kobayashi T, et al. IL-33-responsive lineage- CD25+ CD44 (hi) lymphoid cells mediate innate type 2 immunity and allergic inflammation in the lung. J Immunol. 2012;188:1503–13.
37. Levy BD, De Sanctis GT, Devchand PR, et al. Multi-pronged inhibition of airway hyperresponsiveness and inflammation by lipoxin A4. Nat Med. 2002;9:1018–23.
38. Ilmarinen P, Kankaanranta H. Eosinophil apoptosis as a therapeutic target in allergic asthma. Basic Clin Pharmacol Toxicol. 2014;114:109–17.
39. Zhang X, Moilanen E, Kankaanranta H. Enhancement of human eosinophil apoptosis by fluticasone propionate, budesonide, and beclomethasone. Eur J Pharmacol. 2000;406:325–32.
40. Zhang X, Moilanen E, Adcock IM, et al. Divergent effect of mometasone on human eosinophil and neutrophil apoptosis. Life Sci. 2002;71:1523–34.
41. Molfino NA, Gossage D, Kolbeck R, et al. Molecular and clinical rationale for therapeutic targeting of interleukin-5 and its receptor. Clin Exp Allergy. 2012;42:712–37.
42. Pelaia G, Vatrella A, Maselli R. The potential of biologics for the treatment of asthma. Nat Rev Drug Discov. 2012;11:958–72.
43. Gallelli L, Busceti MT, Vatrella A, et al. Update on anticytokine treatment for asthma. Biomed Res Int. 2013;2013:104315.
44. Newcomb DC, Peebles Jr RS. Th17-mediated inflammation in asthma. Curr Opin Immunol. 2013;25:755–60.

45. Cosmi L, Liotta F, Maggi S, et al. Th17 cells: new players in asthma pathogenesis. Allergy. 2011;66:989–98.
46. Al-Ramli W, Prefontaine D, Chouiali F, et al. T_H17-associated cytokines (IL-17A and IL-17F) in severe asthma. J Allergy Clin Immunol. 2009;123:1185–7.
47. Iezzi G, Sonderegger I, Ampenberger F, et al. CD40-CD40L cross-talk integrates strong antigenic signals and microbial stimuli to induce development of IL-17-producing CD4+ T cells. Proc Natl Acad Sci U S A. 2009;106:876–81.
48. Huang G, Wang Y, Chi H. Regulation of T_H17 cell differentiation by innate immune signals. Cell Mol Immunol. 2012;9:287–95.
49. Bettelli E, Carrier Y, Gao W, et al. Reciprocal developmental pathways for the generation of pathogenic effector T_H17 and regulatory T cells. Nature. 2006;7090:235–8.
50. McGeachy MJ, Chen Y, Tato CM, et al. The interleukin 23 receptor is essential for the terminal differentiation of interleukin 17-producing effector T helper cells in vivo. Nat Immunol. 2009;10:314–24.
51. Thomson NC, Chaudhuri R, Livingston E. Asthma and cigarette smoking. Eur Respir J. 2004;24:822–33.
52. Polosa R, Thomson NC. Smoking and asthma: dangerous liaisons. Eur Respir J. 2013;41:716–26.
53. Brusselle GG, Provoost S, Bracke KR, et al. Inflammasomes in respiratory disease: from bench to bedside. Chest. 2014;145:1121–33.
54. Lee TH, Song HJ, Park CS. Role of inflammasome activation in development and exacerbation of asthma. Asia Pac Allergy. 2014;4:187–96.
55. Ozseker F, Buyukozturk S, Depboylu B, et al. Serum amyloid A (SAA) in induced sputum of asthmatics: a new look to an older marker. Int Immunopharmacol. 2006;6:1569–76.
56. Said-Sadier N, Ojcius DM. Alarmins, inflammasomes and immunity. Biomed J. 2012;35:437–49.
57. Simpson JL, Phipps S, Baines KJ, et al. Elevated expression of the NLRP3 inflammasome in neutrophilic asthma. Eur Respir J. 2014;43:1067–76.
58. Kim HY, Lee HJ, Chang YJ, et al. Interleukin-17-producing innate lymphoid cells and the NLRP3 inflammasome facilitate obesity-associated airway hyper-reactivity. Nat Med. 2014;20:54–61.
59. Manni ML, Robinson KM, Alcorn JF. A tale of two cytokines: IL-17 and IL-22 in asthma and infection. Expert Rev Respir Med. 2014;8:25–42.
60. Serafini N, Klein Wolterink RG, Satoh-Takayama N, et al. Gata3 drives development of RORγt+ group 3 innate lymphoid cells. J Exp Med. 2014;211:199–208.
61. Durrant DM, Metzger DW. Emerging roles of T helper subsets in the pathogenesis of asthma. Immunol Investig. 2010;39:526–49.
62. Wang YH, Wills-Karp MS. The potential role of interleukin-17 in severe asthma. Curr Allergy Asthma Rep. 2011;11:388–94.
63. Halwani R, Al-Muhsen S, Hamid Q. T helper 17 cells in airway diseases: from laboratory bench to bedside. Chest. 2013;143:494–501.
64. Lindén A, Dahlén B. Interleukin-17 cytokine signalling in patients with asthma. Eur Respir J. 2014;44:1319–31.
65. Saffar AS, Ashdown H, Gounni AS. The molecular mechanisms of glucocorticoids-mediated neutrophil survival. Curr Drug Targets. 2011;12:556–62.
66. Kadowaki N. Dendritic cells: a conductor of T cell differentiation. Allergol Int. 2007;56:193–9.
67. Berry MA, Hargadon B, Shelley M, et al. Evidence of a role of tumor necrosis factor α in refractory asthma. N Engl J Med. 2006;354:697–708.
68. Cosmi L, Maggi L, Santarlasci V, et al. Identification of a novel subset of human circulating memory CD4+ T cells that produce both IL-17A and IL-4. J Allergy Clin Immunol. 2010;125:222–30.

69. Irvin C, Zafar I, Good J, et al. Increased frequency of dual-positive T_H2/T_H17 cells in bronchoalveolar lavage fluid characterizes a population of patients with severe asthma. J Allergy Clin Immunol. 2014;134:1175–86.
70. Wang YH, Voo KS, Liu B, et al. A novel subset of CD4(+) T(H)2 memory effector cells that produce inflammatory IL-17 cytokine and promote the exacerbation of chronic allergic asthma. J Exp Med. 2010;207:2479–91.
71. Bhakta NR, Erle DJ. IL-17 and "T_H2-high" asthma: adding fuel to the fire? J Allergy Clin Immunol. 2014;134:1187–8.
72. Jenkins HA, Cherniack R, Szefler SJ, et al. A comparison of the clinical characteristics of children and adults with severe asthma. Chest. 2003;124:1318–24.
73. Wenzel SE. Asthma: defining of the persistent adult phenotypes. Lancet. 2006;368:804–13.
74. Matsumoto K, Inoue H, Fukuyama S, et al. Frequency of Foxp3+CD4+CD25+ T cells is associated with the phenotypes of allergic asthma. Respirology. 2009;14:187–94.
75. Provoost S, Maes T, van Durme YM, et al. Decreased FOXP3 protein expression in patients with asthma. Allergy. 2009;64:1539–46.
76. Palomares O, Martin-Fontecha M, Lauener R, et al. Regulatory T cells and immune regulation of allergic diseases: roles of IL-10 and TGF-β. Genes Immunity. 2014;15:511–20.
77. Lloyd CM, Hessel EM. Functions of T cells in asthma: more than just T_H2 cells. Nat Rev Immunol. 2010;10:838–48.
78. Dougherty RH, Fahy JV. Acute exacerbations of asthma: epidemiology, biology and the exacerbation-prone phenotype. Clin Exp Allergy. 2009;39:193–202.
79. Contoli M, Message SD, Laza-Stanca V, et al. Role of deficient type III interferon-λ production in asthma exacerbations. Nat Med. 2006;12:1023–6.
80. Baraldo S, Contoli M, Bazzan E, et al. Deficient antiviral immune responses in childhood: distinct roles of atopy and asthma. J Allergy Clin Immunol. 2012;130:1307–14.

In addition to chronic inflammation, both allergic and non-allergic phenotypes of asthma are also frequently characterized by dynamic structural changes which involve all layers of the bronchial wall, including large and small airways [1, 2]. Such structural changes, collectively referred as airway remodelling, likely originate from repetitive cycles of tissue injury, causing subsequent cellular responses leading to abnormal repair [3]. Although the concomitance in asthmatic airways of structural modifications and inflammation had previously suggested that the latter could causally determine the development and progression of bronchial remodelling, these two phenomena are currently believed to be quite independent [4, 5]. Indeed, airway remodelling can start during the very initial stages of the natural history of asthma, even at early childhood well before a long-term firm establishment of chronic inflammation [6]. However, close interactions tightly connect the cellular and molecular mechanisms underpinning airway inflammation and remodelling (Fig. 3.1), and both pathologic processes certainly contribute together to induce bronchial hyperresponsiveness as well as asthma persistence and progression, especially in most severe disease phenotypes [7–9].

Overall, airway remodelling in asthma comprises epithelial changes, subepithelial and airway smooth muscle (ASM) thickening as well as bronchial neoangiogenesis (Fig. 3.1).

Epithelial Changes

Within the columnar epithelial layer of human airways, both ciliated and goblet cells undergo relevant structural and functional changes in asthma.

Ciliated epithelial cells of asthmatic bronchi are fragile and vulnerable to tissue injury, and they seem to be intrinsically susceptible to destructive damage and prematurely programmed cell death (apoptosis) [10–15]. Therefore, increased apoptosis can probably contribute in a prominent manner to shape the typical airway surface features, especially detectable in severe asthma, including shedding and denudation of ciliated epithelial cells, which easily detach from basement membrane. Among the several cytokines and growth factors responsible for airway remodelling in asthma, transforming growth factor-β (TGF-β) plays a key pathobiologic role in the apoptotic death of bronchial epithelial cells [15–17]. Indeed, higher levels of TGF-β can be found in the airways of asthmatic patients when compared

© Springer International Publishing Switzerland 2017 17
G. Pelaia et al., *Asthma: Targeted Biological Therapies*,
DOI 10.1007/978-3-319-46007-9_3

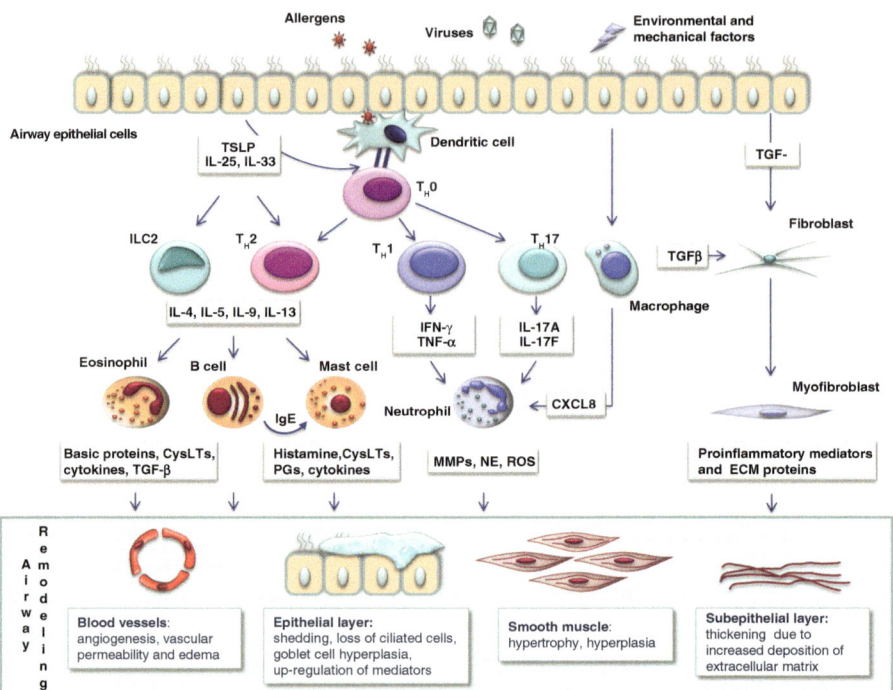

Fig. 3.1 Interactions between airway inflammation and remodelling in asthma. In the pathobiology of asthma, many mediators, cytokines/chemokines, growth factors and enzymes produced by several different cells involved in chronic bronchial inflammation can also affect the functions and proliferation rates of airway structural cells including epithelial cells, fibroblasts/myofibroblasts, smooth muscle cells and endothelial vascular cells

to normal subjects [18, 19]. In asthmatic patients, damaged airway epithelium is one of the main cellular sources of TGF-β, which in turn can act on the same bronchial epithelial cells inducing their apoptosis [16, 20]. Hence, by exerting its pro-apoptotic effect via stimulation of such an autocrine loop, TGF-β perpetuates and amplifies the damage of airway epithelial cells, thereby implementing a vicious pathogenic circuit leading to a self-maintaining tissue destruction especially active in severe asthma. In addition to this autocrine pathway, TGF-β is also produced by inflammatory cells infiltrating asthmatic airways like eosinophils and mast cells [9, 17], which thus further contribute to elicit the apoptosis of bronchial epithelial cells.

A hallmark of airway epithelial remodelling in asthma is represented by hyperplasia/metaplasia of mucus producing goblet cells [21], which are intermixed between columnar ciliated cells. These structural changes span throughout all levels of asthma severity, but they are more prominent in severe and fatal disease [22, 23]. Hyperplastic goblet cells are largely responsible for mucus hypersecretion, which significantly contributes to airway narrowing in asthma. In particular, in asthmatic airways, MUC5AC is the most abundant mucin glycoprotein produced by goblet cells [24]. T-cell-derived type 2 cytokines, and especially IL-13, are powerful inducers of goblet cell hyperplasia and mucus production [25]. In this regard, it is noteworthy that airway goblet cell hyperplasia elicited by IL-13 is steroid resistant [26]. IL-13-dependent goblet cell proliferation and mucus hypersecretion are mediated via overexpression of TGF-β2. Indeed, TGF-β2 levels correlate with mucin expression in asthmatic airways [17, 27]. In addition to the mechanisms activated by IL-13 and TGF-β2, other cellular pathways are implicated in mucin production. In fact, mucus secretion is up-regulated by stimulation of the epidermal growth factor (EGF) receptor, which can be activated by EGF, TGF-α, amphiregulin, epiregulin and β cellulin [24, 28].

Subepithelial Thickening

A major histopathological feature of airway remodelling in asthma, especially occurring in more severe disease, is subepithelial fibrosis [3]. The latter appears at light microscopy as a remarkable thickening of the deepest layer of the basement membrane, called *lamina reticularis* or reticular basement membrane (RBM). Such an increased RBM thickness is primarily due to an enhanced deposition of extracellular matrix (ECM) proteins, including collagens I and III, tenascin, fibronectin and vimentin [29]. The latter are mainly produced by activated fibroblasts and myofibroblasts, stimulated by TGF-β [30]. Accumulation of ECM proteins is markedly favoured by an imbalance between extracellular matrix degrading metalloproteinases (MMPs) and their inhibitors (tissue inhibitors of matrix metalloproteinases—TIMPs). RBM thickening strongly depends on intense communications between airway epithelium and the underlying mesenchyme. In particular, asthmatic airways are characterized by a pathologic reactivation of the epithelial-mesenchymal trophic unit [6], which is physiologically active only during foetal life with the aim of driving lung morphogenesis. Within this pathobiologic context, TGF-β plays a central role by decreasing MMP production and stimulating TIMP synthesis, as well as by promoting the proliferation of bronchial fibroblasts and their differentiation to myofibroblasts [17, 31]. These mesenchymal cells in turn produce high quantities of TGF-β, thereby amplifying the airway fibrotic response in chronic asthma. TGF-β is also synthesized in large amounts by human bronchial epithelium undergoing mechanical stress caused by repetitive cycles of bronchoconstriction [32]. In fact, airway smooth muscle contraction elicited by either inhaled allergens or methacholine enhances TGF-β immunoreactivity within the bronchial epithelium, thus increasing the thickness of the subepithelial collagen sheet [33]. These findings, obtained in asthmatic patients, have thereby corroborated the results of previous in vitro experiments, showing that compression of airway epithelial cells induced the production of collagens I, III and IV by cocultured bronchial fibroblasts [34].

In addition to TGF-β, other cytokines, and especially those released by Th2 lymphocytes, markedly contribute to induce airway subepithelial remodelling in asthma [9]. For instance, by promoting the differentiation, recruitment, activation and survival of eosinophils, IL-5 also stimulates eosinophil synthesis of TGF-β. In this regard, IL-5-deficient mice repeatedly exposed to allergen challenge were characterized by less prominent peribronchiolar fibrosis and lower numbers of TGF-β-positive cells when compared to wild-type animals [35]. Furthermore, in asthmatic patients, anti-IL-5 biological therapies significantly decreased the bronchial production of subepithelial ECM proteins, such as procollagen III, tenascin and lumican, and also reduced BAL levels of TGF-β1, as well as the numbers of TGF-β1-positive eosinophils [36, 37]. Other Th2 cytokines which are involved in the pathogenesis of airway subepithelial fibrosis in asthma are IL-4 and especially IL-13 [38]. The latter up-regulates the synthesis of ECM proteins and promotes the phenotypic transition from lung fibroblasts to myofibroblasts [39]: these effects are at least in part mediated by periostin, a multifunctional matricellular protein expressed in the airways by both inflammatory and structural cells. Indeed, acting together with TGF-β, IL-4 and IL-13 stimulate bronchial fibroblasts to produce periostin, which in turn implements autocrine mechanisms leading to an increased synthesis of ECM proteins, as well as to fibroblast differentiation into myofibroblasts [40].

Airway Smooth Muscle Remodelling

The increased thickness of airway smooth muscle (ASM) layer is one of the main factors contributing to bronchial remodelling and hyperreactivity in asthma. Indeed, the amount of ASM mass appears to be directly correlated to both duration and severity of asthma, as well as to airway hyperresponsiveness to methacholine [8, 41–43]. In patients with asthma, and particularly in those subjects suffering from more severe disease, the oversized ASM bundle arises from an enlargement of ASM cell volume (cellular hypertrophy) and especially from ASM cell proliferation (cellular hyperplasia) [44, 45]. An important mechanism which induces ASM hypertrophy is the mechanical stretch consequent to persistent bronchoconstriction [46]. However, with respect to ASM hypertrophy, much more information is currently available about ASM hyperplasia.

An increased proliferation of ASM cells has been shown in both asthmatic patients and animal models of allergic airway inflammation [47, 48]. ASM mitogens include growth factors, contractile agonists and perhaps pro-inflammatory cytokines. Among the first ones, a relevant proliferative action is exerted by TGF-β, EGF, insulin-like growth factors (IGFs), platelet-derived growth factor (PDGF) and fibroblast growth factor-2 (FGF-2). Interestingly, some of the agents that induce ASM contraction, such as histamine, endothelin-1, substance P, serotonin, α-thrombin, thromboxane A_2 and leukotriene D_4 (LTD$_4$), are also able to behave as mitogenic stimuli [49]. Furthermore, in ASM derived from asthmatic patients, when compared to normal subjects, low levels have been found of the bronchodilating prostaglandin E_2 (PGE$_2$) [50], which is also an inhibitor of ASM cell growth [51]. More controversial is the potential proliferative role of inflammatory cytokines like IL-1β, IL-6, and TNF-α, whose mitogenic actions have been shown in ASM of some animal species [52]. Moreover, IL-13 is able in vitro to potentiate the proliferative effects induced by LTD$_4$ on human ASM [53].

Once again, in asthmatic airways, TGF-β plays a prominent role also with regard to ASM remodelling. In fact, TGF-β can be secreted by ASM cells, which also express TGF-β receptors [17]. TGF-β stimulates ASM proliferation either directly via an autocrine loop or also indirectly by inducing the production of connective tissue growth factor (CTGF), which is a powerful ASM mitogen [54]. Moreover, TGF-β exerts on ASM a synergistic proliferative action with FGF-2 and is also capable of eliciting an anti-apoptotic effect on ASM cells [55]. In addition to cytokines and growth factors, ECM proteins are also implicated in ASM proliferation [44]. In this regard, it is noteworthy that ASM cells obtained from asthmatic patients express relevant changes in their secretory profile of matrix proteins, which is characterized by an increased production of fibulin 1-C, capable of enhancing proliferation of asthmatic ASM [56, 57].

A further demonstration of the clinical and functional relevance of ASM remodelling in asthma can be inferred from the significant benefits achievable by severe asthmatic patients undergoing a hyperthermic treatment of airways with radiofrequency waves (bronchial thermoplasty), performed via bronchoscopy, and aimed to decrease ASM bulk. In particular, several studies have shown that bronchial thermoplasty is a safe procedure which reduces ASM mass in subjects with severe asthma, thus lowering bronchial hyperresponsiveness, annual rates of disease exacerbations and utilization of healthcare services [58, 59].

Increased Bronchial Vasculature

Both qualitative and quantitative changes characterize the airway microcirculation in asthma [60, 61]. These alterations, leading to an increased bronchial blood flow and contributing to the enhanced thickness of asthmatic airway walls, include vasodilatation and neoangiogenesis. The latter, resulting from growth of new blood vessels, is the predominant feature of the bronchial vascular remodelling occurring in asthma. In particular, the most important mechanism underlying the enlargement of airway vascular area in asthma is endothelial cell proliferation [62]. Among the angiogenic agents responsible for the increased numbers of arterioles and capillaries detectable in asthmatic bronchi, vascular endothelial growth factor (VEGF) plays the most relevant pathogenic role [63]. VEGF is overexpressed in the airways of patients with asthma, and this potent vascular growth factor is produced not only by endothelial cells but also by many inflammatory cells such as eosinophils, macrophages and mast cells [64, 65]. In addition to VEGF, angiopoietin-1 (Ang-1) is another vascular growth factor which induces neovascularization in asthma [61]. Relatively high amounts of both VEGF and Ang-1 have been found in the induced sputum from patients with severe asthma [65, 66]. Indeed, although a relevant vascular component of airway remodelling can be detected even in patients with mild-to-moderate asthma, however, some studies suggest that a relationship may exist between disease severity and the amplitude of the bronchial area occupied by blood vessels [67, 68].

Concluding Remarks

Together with airway inflammation, bronchial remodelling is a major pathologic feature of chronic asthma. Although airway inflammation and remodelling affect each other by reciprocal intercellular communications involving a complex network of cytokines and growth factors (Fig. 3.1), structural changes can occur independently of inflammation and may even precede the onset of asthma symptoms [69]. Hallmarks of airway remodelling in asthma include epithelial shedding and goblet cell hyperplasia, subepithelial fibrosis with abnormal deposition of extracellular matrix, enhanced thickness of smooth muscle layer and neoangiogenesis of bronchial vasculature (Fig. 3.1) [8]. Airway remodelling could provide some potential benefits in asthma, in that an increased stiffness might enable the airways to resist dynamic compression; furthermore, deposition of collagen fibres around ASM could produce a mechanical impedance to contraction. Nevertheless, these theoretical advantages are largely overcome by the negative effects of remodelling, which results in narrowing of the bronchial lumen and fixed airway obstruction, with impaired response to bronchodilators [69]. Such aspects largely predominate in patients with severe asthma, who are often characterized by poorly reversible airflow limitation and progressive decline of lung function [70].

References

1. Jeffery PK. Remodeling in asthma and chronic obstructive pulmonary disease. Am J Respir Crit Care Med. 2001;164:S28–38.
2. Turato G, Barbato A, Baraldo S, et al. Nonatopic children with multitrigger wheezing have airway pathology comparable to atopic asthma. Am J Respir Crit Care Med. 2008;178:476–82.
3. Trejo Bittar HE, Yousem SA, Wenzel SE. Pathobiology of severe asthma. Annu Rev Pathol. 2015;10:511–45.
4. Homer RJ, Elias JA. Airway remodeling in asthma: therapeutic implications of mechanisms. Physiology. 2005;20:28–35.
5. Hirota N, Martin JG. Mechanisms of airway remodeling. Chest. 2013;144:1026–32.
6. Holgate ST, Holloway J, Wilson S, et al. Epithelial-mesenchymal communication in the pathogenesis of chronic asthma. Proc Am Thorac Soc. 2004;1:93–8.
7. Cohn L, Elias JA, Chupp GL. Asthma: mechanisms of disease persistence and progression. Annu Rev Immunol. 2004;22:789–815.
8. Pascual RM, Peters SP. Airway remodeling contributes to the progressive loss of lung function in asthma: an overview. J Allergy Clin Immunol. 2005;116:477–86.
9. Doherty T, Broide D. Cytokines and growth factors in airway remodeling in asthma. Curr Opin Immunol. 2007;19:676–80.
10. Druilhe A, Wallaert B, Tsicopoulos A, et al. Apoptosis, proliferation, and expression of Bcl-2, Fas, and Fas ligand in bronchial biopsies from asthmatics. Am J Respir Cell Mol Biol. 1998;19:747–57.
11. Benayoun L, Letuve A, Druilhe J, et al. Regulation of peroxisome proliferator-activated receptor gamma expression in human asthmatic airways; relationship with proliferation, apoptosis, and airway remodeling. Am J Respir Crit Care Med. 2001;164:1487–94.
12. Trautmann AP, Schmid-Grendelmeier K, Kruger R, et al. T cells and eosinophils cooperate in the induction of bronchial epithelial cell apoptosis in asthma. J Allergy Clin Immunol. 2002;109:329–37.

13. Bucchieri F, Puddicombe SM, Lordan JL, et al. Asthmatic bronchial epithelium is more susceptible to oxidant-induced apoptosis. Am J Respir Cell Mol Biol. 2002;27:179–85.
14. Cohen L, Xueping E, Tarsi J, et al. Epithelial cell proliferation contributes to airway remodeling in severe asthma. Am J Respir Crit Care Med. 2007;176:138–45.
15. O'Sullivan MP, Tyner JW, Holtzman MJ. Apoptosis in the airways: another balancing act in the epithelial program. Am J Respir Cell Mol Biol. 2003;29:3–7.
16. Pelaia G, Cuda G, Vatrella A, et al. Effects of transforming growth factor-β and budesonide on mitogen-activated protein kinase activation and apoptosis in airway epithelial cells. Am J Respir Cell Mol Biol. 2003;29:12–8.
17. Makinde T, Murphy RF, Agrawall DK. The regulatory role of TGF-β in airway remodeling in asthma. Immunol Cell Biol. 2007;85:348–56.
18. Redington AE, Madden AJ, Frew R, et al. Transforming growth factor-β1 in asthma: measurement in bronchoalveolar lavage. Am J Respir Crit Care Med. 1997;156:642–7.
19. Hastie AT, Kraft WK, Nyce KB, et al. Asthmatic epithelial cell proliferation and stimulation of collagen production. Am J Respir Crit Care Med. 2002;165:266–72.
20. Vignola AM, Chanez P, Chiappara G, et al. Transforming growth factor-β expression in mucosal biopsies in asthma and chronic bronchitis. Am J Respir Crit Care Med. 1997;156:591–9.
21. Fahy JV. Goblet cell and mucin gene abnormality in asthma. Chest. 2002;122:320S–6.
22. Ordonez CL, Khashayar R, Wong HH, et al. Mild and moderate asthma is associated with airway goblet cell hyperplasia and abnormalities in mucin gene expression. Am J Respir Crit Care Med. 2001;163:517–23.
23. Jenkins HA, Cool C, Szefler SJ, et al. Histopathology of severe childhood asthma: a case series. Chest. 2003;124:32–41.
24. Rubin BK, Priftis KN, Schmidt HJ, et al. Secretory hyperresponsiveness and pulmonary mucus hypersecretion. Chest. 2014;146:496–507.
25. Fahy JV, Dickey BF. Airway mucus function and dysfunction. N Engl J Med. 2010;363:2233–47.
26. Kanoh S, Tanabe T, Rubin BK. IL-13-induced MUC5AC production and goblet cell differentiation is steroid resistant in human airway cells. Clin Exp Allergy. 2011;41:1747–56.
27. Chu HW, Balzar S, Seedorf GJ, et al. Transforming growth factor-β2 induces bronchial epithelial mucin expression in asthma. Am J Pathol. 2004;165:1097–106.
28. Burgel PR, Nadel JA. Role of epidermal growth factor receptor activation in epithelial cell repair and mucin production in airway epithelium. Thorax. 2004;59:992–6.
29. Jeffery PK, Laitinen A, Venge P. Biopsy markers of airway inflammation and remodelling. Respir Med. 2000;94(Suppl F):S9–15.
30. Knight D. Epithelium-fibroblast interactions in response to airway inflammation. Immunol Cell Biol. 2001;79:160–4.
31. Wynn TA. Common and unique mechanisms regulate fibrosis in various fibroproliferative diseases. J Clin Invest. 2007;117:524–9.
32. Gosens R, Grainge C. Bronchoconstriction and airway biology – potential impact and therapeutic opportunities. Chest. 2015;147:798–803.
33. Grainge CL, Lau LCK, Ward JA, et al. Effect of bronchoconstriction on airway remodeling in asthma. N Engl J Med. 2011;364:2006–15.
34. Swartz MA, Tschumperlin DJ, Kamm RD, et al. Mechanical stress is communicated between different cell types to elicit matrix remodeling. Proc Natl Acad Sci U S A. 2001;98:6180–5.
35. Cho JY, Miller M, Baek KJ, et al. Inhibition of airway remodeling in IL-5 deficient mice. J Clin Invest. 2004;113:551–60.
36. Flood-Page P, Menzies-Gow A, Phipps S, et al. Anti-IL-5 treatment reduces deposition of ECM proteins in the bronchial subepithelial basement membrane of mild atopic asthmatics. J Clin Invest. 2003;112:1029–36.
37. Humbles AA, Lloyd CM, McMillan SJ, et al. A critical role for eosinophils in allergic airways remodeling. Science. 2004;305:1776–9.
38. Doucet C, Brouty-Boye D, Pottin-Clemenceau C, et al. Interleukin (IL) 4 and IL-13 act on human lung fibroblasts. Implication in asthma. J Clin Invest. 1998;101:2129–39.

39. Hashimoto S, Gon Y, Takeshita I, et al. IL-4 and IL-13 induce myofibroblastic phenotype of human lung fibroblasts through c-Jun NH$_2$-terminal kinase-dependent pathway. J Allergy Clin Immunol. 2001;107:1001–8.
40. Li W, Gao P, Zhi Y. Periostin: its role in asthma and its potential as a diagnostic or therapeutic target. Respir Res. 2015;16:57.
41. Bai TR, Cooper J, Koelmeyer T, et al. The effect of age and duration of disease on airway structure in fatal asthma. Am J Respir Crit Care Med. 2000;162:663–9.
42. Pepe C, Foley S, Shannon J, et al. Differences in airway remodeling between subjects with severe and moderate asthma. J Allergy Clin Immunol. 2005;116:544–9.
43. Sapienza S, Du T, Eidelman DH, et al. Structural changes in the airways of sensitised brown Norway rats after antigen challenge. Am Rev Respir Dis. 1991;144:423–7.
44. Black JL, Panettieri Jr RA, Banerjee A, et al. Airway smooth muscle in asthma – just a target for Bronchodilation? Clin Chest Med. 2012;33:543–58.
45. James AL, Elliot JG, Jones RL, et al. Airway smooth muscle hypertrophy and hyperplasia in asthma. Am J Respir Crit Care Med. 2012;185:1058–64.
46. Tschumperlin DJ, Drazen JM. Mechanical stimuli to airway remodeling. Am J Respir Crit Care Med. 2001;164:S90–4.
47. Johnson PR, Roth M, Tamm M, et al. Airway smooth muscle cell proliferation is increased in asthma. Am J Respir Crit Care Med. 2001;164:474–7.
48. Hirst SJ, Martin JG, Bonacci JV, et al. Proliferative aspects of airway smooth muscle. J Allergy Clin Immunol. 2004;114(2 Suppl):S2–17.
49. Pelaia G, Renda T, Gallelli L, et al. Molecular mechanisms underlying airway smooth muscle contraction and proliferation: implications for asthma. Respir Med. 2008;102:1173–81.
50. Chambers LS, Black JL, Ge Q, et al. PAR-2 activation, PGE2, and COX-2 in human asthmatic and nonasthmatic airway smooth muscle cells. Am J Physiol Lung Cell Mol Physiol. 2003;285:L619–27.
51. Belvisi MG, Saunders M, Yacoub M, et al. Expression of cyclo-oxygenase-2 in human airway smooth muscle is associated with profound reductions in cell growth. Br J Pharmacol. 1998;125:1102–8.
52. Lazaar AL, Panettieri RA. Airway smooth muscle as a regulator of immune responses and bronchomotor tone. Clin Chest Med. 2006;27:53–69.
53. Espinosa K, Bossé Y, Stankova J, et al. Cys-LT1 receptor upregulation by TGF-β and IL-13 is associated with bronchial smooth muscle cell proliferation in response to LTD4. J Allergy Clin Immunol. 2003;111:1032–40.
54. Chen G, Khalil N. TGF-β1 increases proliferation of airway smooth muscle cells by phosphorylation of map kinases. Respir Res. 2006;7:2.
55. Bosse Y, Thompson C, Stankova J, et al. Fibroblast growth factor 2 and transforming growth factor β1 synergism in human bronchial smooth muscle cell proliferation. Am J Respir Cell Mol Biol. 2006;34:746–53.
56. Johnson PR, Burgess JK, Underwood PA, et al. Extracellular matrix proteins modulate asthmatic airway smooth muscle cell proliferation via an autocrine mechanism. J Allergy Clin Immunol. 2004;113:690–6.
57. Lau JY, Oliver BG, Baraket M, et al. Fibulin-1 is increased in asthma – a novel mediator of airway remodeling? PLoS One. 2010;5:e13360.
58. Cox G, Miller JD, McWilliams A, et al. Bronchial thermoplasty for asthma. Am J Respir Crit Care Med. 2006;173:965–9.
59. Laxmanan B, Hogarth DK. Bronchial thermoplasty in asthma: current perspectives. J Asthma Allergy. 2015;8:39–49.
60. Salvato G. Quantitative and morphologic analysis of the vascular bed in bronchial biopsy specimens from asthmatic and non-asthmatic subjects. Thorax. 2001;56:902–6.
61. Chetta A, Zanini A, Torre O, et al. Vascular remodeling and angiogenesis in asthma: morphological aspects and pharmacological modulation. Inflamm Allergy Drug Targets. 2006;6:41–5.

62. McDonald DM. Angiogenesis and remodeling of airway vasculature in chronic inflammation. Am J Respir Crit Care Med. 2001;164:S39–45.
63. Hoshino M, Takahashi M, Aoike N. Expression of vascular endothelial growth factor, basic fibroblast growth factor and angiogenin immunoreactivity in asthmatic airways ant its relationships to angiogenesis. J Allergy Clin Immunol. 2001;107:295–301.
64. Chetta A, Zanini A, Foresi A, et al. Vascular endothelial growth factor up-regulation and bronchial wall remodelling in asthma. Clin Exp Allergy. 2005;35:1437–42.
65. Tseliou E, Bakakos P, Kostikas K, et al. Increased levels of angiopoietin 1 and 2 in sputum supernatant in severe refractory asthma. Allergy. 2012;67:396–402.
66. Papadaki G, Bakakos P, Kostikas K, et al. Vascular endothelial growth factor and cysteinyl leukotrienes in sputum supernatant of patients with asthma. Respir Med. 2013;107:1339–45.
67. Hashimoto M, Tanaka H, Abe S. Quantitative analysis of bronchial wall vascularity in the medium and small airways of patients with asthma and COPD. Chest. 2005;127:965–72.
68. Vrugt B, Wilson S, Bron A, et al. Bronchial angiogenesis in severe glucocorticoid-dependent asthma. Eur Respir J. 2000;15:1014–21.
69. Tang MLK, Wilson JW, Stewart AG, et al. Airway remodelling in asthma: current understanding and implications for future therapies. Pharmacol Ther. 2006;112:474–88.
70. Wenzel S. Severe asthma: from characteristics to phenotypes to endotypes. Clin Exp Allergy. 2012;42:650–8.

Anti-IgE Therapy

4

The propensity to develop an exaggerated antibody response to inhaled antigens operated by immunoglobulin E (IgE), which is defined as atopy, plays a central role in the pathobiology of allergic asthma [1]. The pleiotropic effects of IgE are mediated by activation of specific IgE receptors expressed by both immune-inflammatory and airway structural cells [2–4]. IgE were identified in 1967 by Ishizaka and Ishizaka, and since then these antibodies have been considered as suitable molecular targets for the development of anti-allergy therapies [5, 6]. However, it took almost 40 years to translate this key immunological discovery into the approval of the anti-IgE antibody omalizumab for the treatment of severe allergic asthma [7]. Indeed, omalizumab has been the first and for a long time the only biologic drug available in clinical practice for add-on therapy of uncontrolled asthma [8].

Role of IgE in Allergic Asthma

In atopic asthmatic patients, IgE are synthesized in lymph nodes and airway mucosa by lymphocytes B upon IL-4-induced Ig class switching, consisting of a complex antibody recombination resulting in the prevalent production of IgE [9, 10]. The molecular structure of IgE is made of two variable antigen-binding fragments (Fab) and a receptor-binding constant portion (Fc). In particular, the IgE molecule (molecular weight, 190 kD) comprises two identical light chains, each including a variable (V_L) and a constant domain (C_L), as well as two identical heavy chains, each constituted by a single-domain variable region (V_H) and a constant region containing four domains (Cε1, Cε2, Cε3, Cε4). The biologic functions of IgE depend on binding of their two Cε3 domains to high-affinity (FcεRI) and low-affinity (FcεRII/CD23) IgE receptors located in the plasma membrane of several target cells.

FcεRI are expressed as $\alpha\beta\gamma_2$ tetramers on mast cells and basophils and as $\alpha\gamma_2$ trimers on monocytes/macrophages, eosinophils, myeloid and plasmacytoid dendritic cells, as well as on resident cells such as bronchial epithelial cells and airway smooth muscle cells [2, 4, 11, 12]. FcεRI interact with IgE through the two extracellular domains of their α chain, which bind the two Cε3 domains of IgE, whereas the intracellular β and γ chains are involved in signal transduction. X-ray crystallographic studies have shown that, as a consequence of the interaction between FcεRI α chain and the two Cε3 domains of IgE, the Cε2 domains fold back asymmetrically, thereby making contacts with both Cε3 and Cε4 domains and causing a

© Springer International Publishing Switzerland 2017   27
G. Pelaia et al., *Asthma: Targeted Biological Therapies*,
DOI 10.1007/978-3-319-46007-9_4

structural bending of IgE molecule [13]; such remarkable conformational changes of IgE structure result in a relevant prolongation of the half-life of IgE receptor complexes. At the level of mast cell and basophil surfaces, adjacent allergenic epitopes induce the aggregation of two or more FcεRI-bound IgE molecules (cross linking), and this event is essential for cell activation. In particular, receptor dimerization activates the FcεRI β subunit-linked protein kinase LYN, which phosphorylates tyrosine residues situated within the cytoplasmic immunoreceptor tyrosine-based activation motif (ITAM) regions of FcεRI β and γ chains [14]. Phosphorylated ITAM regions in turn engage the tyrosine kinase spleen tyrosine kinase (SYK). The following SYK- and/or LYN-mediated tyrosine phosphorylation of the transmembrane adaptor molecule linker for activation of T cells (LAT) coordinates the complex network of downstream signalling pathways which are required for mast cell secretion of various pro-inflammatory mediators [15]. Indeed, LAT phosphorylation results in recruitment and activation of many other adaptor molecules and enzymes [16]. Among the latter, phospholipase Cγ_1 (PLCγ_1) generates diacylglycerol which activates protein kinase C (PKC), responsible for mast cell degranulation and the subsequent release of preformed granule-associated mediators (histamine, tryptase, chymase and heparin). In addition, the parallel RAS-/RAF-dependent stimulation of the mitogen-activated protein kinase (MAPK) family of signalling enzymes leads to phospholipase A$_2$ (PLA$_2$)-catalyzed production of the precursors of newly formed eicosanoids (cysteinyl leukotrienes C$_4$-D$_4$ and prostaglandin D$_2$), as well as to transcription factor-mediated expression of several different cytokines, chemokines and growth factors (IL-3, IL-4, IL-5, IL-6, IL-8, IL-13, RANTES, GM-CSF). These mechanisms are responsible for both early and late responses experienced by atopic asthmatic subjects upon allergen exposure [17]. The early-phase asthmatic response, which takes place within minutes of antigen linkage to FcεRI-bound IgE attached to cell membrane, is mostly due to airway smooth muscle contraction induced by bronchoconstrictive mediators released from mast cells. The late-phase asthmatic response, usually occurring several hours after allergen inhalation, is characterized by bronchoconstriction and inflammatory changes mainly caused by cytokines and chemokines leading to eosinophil activation and recruitment within the airways. Although all these cellular events are predominantly elicited by allergen-dependent IgE dimerization, mast cell activation can also be triggered by monomeric IgE molecules, independently of allergen cross linking. Indeed, human monomeric IgE are able to induce histamine and leukotriene secretion from mast cells and also to prolong their survival via an autocrine production of IL-6 [18, 19]; these effects are further enhanced by mast cell exposure to IL-4 [20].

Low-affinity IgE receptors, named FcεRII or CD23, are characterized by a C-type (calcium-dependent) lectin structure containing a globular IgE-binding domain, associated with a long stalk component which coordinates the assembly of a trimeric receptor complex displaying a barely lower affinity for IgE with respect to high-affinity FcεRI receptors [21, 22]. Two variants of FcεRII receptors exist, originating by alternative splicing of the CD23 gene, which are called CD23a and CD23b, respectively. CD23a is constitutively expressed by B lymphocytes, whereas

CD23b expression on many cell types, including antigen-presenting cells, eosinophils and human bronchial epithelial cells, is stimulated by IL-4 [22, 23].

IgE exert relevant actions with regard to regulation of both FcεRI and FcεRII receptors. In particular, IgE-deficient mice are characterized by low densities of FcεRI and FcεRII on mast cells/basophils and B lymphocytes, respectively; cell membrane expression of both high-affinity and low-affinity receptors can be reintegrated by IgE supplementation [24–26]. These findings have been also confirmed in humans, who exhibit a direct relationship between total serum IgE levels and FcεRI membrane density. In fact, unoccupied receptors undergo internalization, whilst IgE-bound receptors remain on plasma membrane because of an IgE-mediated effective protection against internalization and subsequent proteolytic cleavage [27, 28]. IgE-mediated up-regulation of FcεRI makes mast cells more susceptible to allergenic stimuli which thus become able to induce, even at low concentrations, the release of high amounts of pro-inflammatory agents [25]. Therefore, the progressively increasing numbers of membrane FcεRI receptors contribute to implement a positive, self-maintaining circuit which markedly amplifies the allergic cascade. Moreover, an up-regulation of FcεRI density at level of both mast cells and basophils is elicited by monomeric IgE, in the absence of allergen cross linking [29]. Similarly to mast cells and basophils, FcεRI expression on monocytes and dendritic cells is correlated with IgE blood concentrations, and receptor numbers are increased in atopic subjects [30, 31]. Furthermore, the interaction of IgE with FcεRII/CD23 receptors is able to inhibit their proteolytic degradation, thereby facilitating the stabilization of the IgE-FcεRII complex on cell membrane [32]. By contrast, empty FcεRII easily undergo proteolytic degradation [33], resulting in the release of free receptors named soluble CD23 (sCD23), which maintain the ability to ligate IgE. In addition to sCD23, at least two other human soluble IgE receptors such as soluble FcεRI (sFcεRI) and galectin-3 have been identified [34]. Indeed, besides membrane FcεRI and FcεRII, the existence of soluble IgE receptors is also well known. sFcεRI consists of a single-receptor subunit corresponding to an incomplete variant of the FcεRI α chain [35], which in vitro can be obtained after IgE-dependent aggregation of membrane trimeric FcεRI expressed by antigen-presenting cells [34]. Although the cellular elements which release this receptor protein in vivo have not been precisely identified, sFcεRI is present in human bloodstream where it can ligate the constant region of circulating IgE, thereby preventing these antibodies from binding to membrane-anchored FcεRI [36]. sCD23 can originate by either proteolytic cleavage of FcεRII present on B-cell membrane or intracellular processing of newly synthesized FcεRII receptors, which are subsequently released within exosomes or as free molecules [33, 37, 38]. Both membrane and soluble FcεRII/CD23 receptors are involved in homeostasis of human IgE [39]. In particular, IgE binding to membrane CD23 decreases IgE synthesis, whilst sCD23 enhances IgE production via co-aggregation of cell surface IgE and CD21, which is an additional CD23 ligand [21]. Intracellular galectin-3 is located in the cytosol or in the nucleus of many cell types such as dendritic cells and macrophages; the latter represent the main source of extracellular soluble galectin-3. Upon stimulation by IL-4 and IL-13, macrophages increase galectin-3 secretion [40]. Secreted galectin-3 binds to several extracellular matrix proteins and cell surface molecules, also including IgE and FcεRI [41, 42]. Therefore, galectin-3 can contribute to mast cell/basophil activation by promoting the cross linking of receptor-bound IgE, FcεRI or both [43].

In addition to mast cell-dependent early and late asthmatic reactions, induced by IgE binding to FcεRI, many other pathobiologic events in asthma are mediated by both FcεRI and FcεRII at level of several immune-inflammatory and airway structural cells.

With regard to the functions of dendritic cells, activation of their membrane FcεRI receptors plays a crucial role in allergen uptake, processing and presentation, thereby significantly contributing to antigen-dependent T-cell responses [1, 2, 44]. Indeed, IgE-FcεRI-mediated allergen presentation can critically lower the threshold of atopic subjects in order to mount an allergen-specific activation of T lymphocytes. Furthermore, the IgE-FcεRI interaction occurring on dendritic cell surface also induces the production of CCL28, a chemokine that selectively attracts and activates Th2 cells through binding to their CCR10 receptors [45, 46]. Moreover, IgE-dependent stimulation of FcεRI expressed by plasmacytoid dendritic cells suppresses their synthesis of antiviral interferons, and this effect is mediated by the involvement of ILT7, an inhibitory receptor bearing an ITAM-based activation motif [47].

Eosinophils express FcεRI and FcεRII/CD23 receptors [48–50]. In atopic subjects with airway eosinophilia, FcεRI are located on cell membrane of both blood eosinophils and tissue eosinophils. In human eosinophils, FcεRI can be expressed as either tetrameric or trimeric complexes. A high expression of both FcεRI and FcεRII receptors appears to be associated with eosinophil recruitment. Furthermore, IgE inhibit the apoptotic death of eosinophils, thereby working as survival factors for these cells [51].

Among airway structural cells, IgE receptors are expressed by bronchial epithelial cells, as well as by smooth muscle cells. Expression of both FcεRI and FcεRII/ CD23 receptors has been detected in bronchial epithelial cells [11, 23]. FcεRII work as transporters of IgE or IgE-allergen complexes across the polarized respiratory mucosa [52, 53]. It is thus possible that IgE produced by local B cells interact with their low-affinity receptors on the apical membrane of bronchial epithelial cells and are then released into the airway lumen, where such antibodies can bind inhaled allergens and form antigen/IgE immune complexes. The latter could be transported in the opposite direction towards intraepithelial dendritic cells and mucosal mast cells, thus promoting antigen presentation to Th lymphocytes and mediator release, respectively. These mechanisms might play a key role in initiation and development of airway allergic inflammation because bronchial epithelial cells, given their peculiar position placed at the interface between the respiratory tract and the external environment, are the first cellular elements which come in contact with inhaled allergens. Moreover, it is also possible that IgE stimulate bronchial epithelial cells to synthesize and release growth factors involved in airway remodelling, such as transforming growth factor-β (TGF-β).

FcεRI have also been detected on the surface of airway smooth muscle cells [54]. In asthmatic patients, IgE-dependent activation of airway smooth muscle cell FcεRI could be involved in several effector functions, implicated in cell proliferation as well as in the synthesis of pro-inflammatory mediators and extracellular matrix proteins. In regard to such a latter aspect, it is noteworthy that IgE have been shown to stimulate airway smooth muscle cell production of collagens I and III [55], and this effect could thus significantly contribute to the pathogenesis of bronchial remodelling in asthma.

Omalizumab: Mechanism of Action and Pharmacokinetics

Omalizumab is a recombinant humanized antibody consisting of a human IgG structure that includes specific anti-human IgE determinants of murine origin [56]. As a result of this recombinant technology, only 5 % or less of omalizumab is composed of murine residues, and such structural characteristics are thus associated with a minimal risk of immune responses towards non-self antigenic components [57]. Omalizumab specifically interacts with the two Cε3 domains of IgE, thereby generating either trimeric or hexameric IgE/anti-IgE immune complexes (Fig. 4.1)

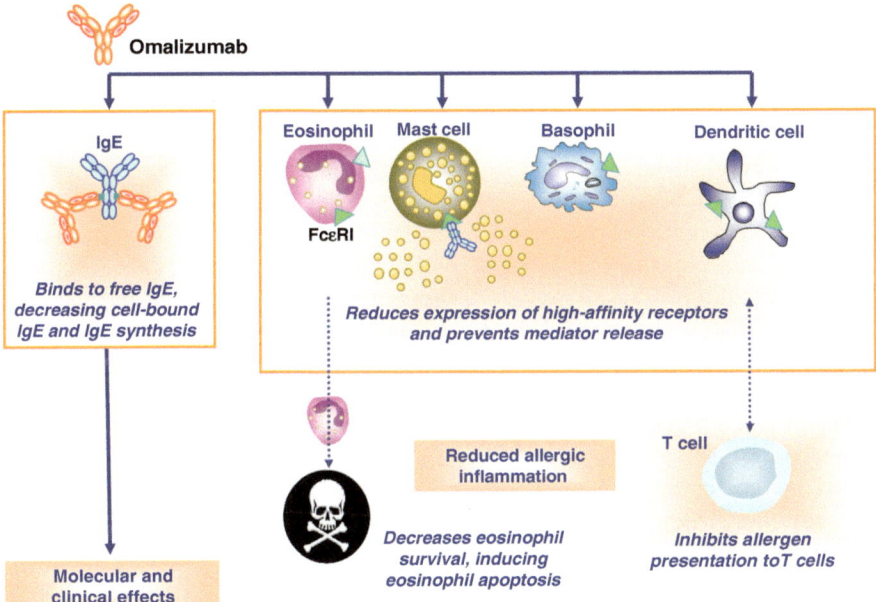

Fig. 4.1 Mechanism of action and cellular targets of omalizumab. Omalizumab binds to and reduces the levels of free IgE, thus inhibiting their binding to cellular receptors expressed by mast cells, basophils, eosinophils and dendritic cells. As a consequence, IgE-dependent antigen presentation to T-helper cells and allergic responses are inhibited. Anti-IgE therapy with omalizumab also results in decreased FcεRI expression and increased eosinophil apoptosis. All these effects are responsible for a reduction of immune airway inflammation, as well as of the related respiratory symptoms (Reprinted from Ref. [134])

[58]. The small size of such IgE/anti-IgE aggregates guarantees a high safety profile, because these immune complexes are very soluble, do not bind complement and do not precipitate, thus being easily removed by the reticuloendothelial system [58, 59]. Furthermore, because of the high affinity of omalizumab for IgE, IgE/omalizumab immune complexes are very stable and do not diffuse through vascular walls, thus accumulating within the sites where they assemble, namely, inside blood vessels or in local tissues such as airways and nasal mucosa [60].

Since omalizumab binds to the Cε3 domain, which is the common site where FcεRI and FcεRII/CD23 interact with IgE, this monoclonal antibody is capable of inhibiting the pathobiologic events mediated by activation of both high-affinity and low-affinity receptors [60, 61]. Therefore, by impeding IgE linkage to FcεRI, omalizumab prevents allergen-dependent IgE dimerization and the subsequent degranulation of mast cells and basophils (Fig. 4.1), as well as the secretion of lipid mediators and the production of cytokines/chemokines elicited by FcεRI activation induced by IgE. Furthermore, it has been suggested that omalizumab can also interfere with mast cell functions independently of inhibition of IgE dimerization. In particular, omalizumab could prevent the direct effects promoted by monomeric IgE/FcεRI interactions on intracellular mast cell signalling pathways, whose activation leads to an increased synthesis of cytokines such as IL-4, IL-6, IL-13 and tumour necrosis factor-α (TNF-α), as well as to a prolonged mast cell survival [29, 62]. Hence, by inhibiting the synthesis of cytokines and growth factors essential for survival of mast cells, omalizumab can induce mast cell apoptosis. Similarly, this drug also elicits eosinophil apoptosis. Indeed, omalizumab enhances eosinophil staining for the apoptotic marker annexin V, and this action is due to a reduced production of eosinophil survival factors, such as granulocyte-macrophage colony-stimulating factor (GM-CSF) [63].

Omalizumab-induced blockade of IgE/FcεRI interactions also decreases by about 97 % basophil FcεRI expression, and this reduction is associated with lower responses of mast cells and basophils to allergen stimulation [57]. Indeed, due to the very low availability of free IgE molecules in the presence of omalizumab, unoccupied FcεRI receptors located on basophil cell membrane can be internalized inside the cytoplasm, without being resynthesized [62]. When omalizumab ligates serum IgE, their free levels in peripheral blood decrease by 96–99 % [64]. Moreover, by impeding IgE interactions with FcεRI located on the surface of dendritic cells (Fig. 4.1), omalizumab significantly attenuates the process of antigen presentation to T cells. Omalizumab can also repress IgE synthesis, and this effect is likely mediated by inhibition of IgE binding to FcεRII receptors located on IgE-producing B lymphocytes. Another action of omalizumab, possibly also involved in decreasing IgE expression, can be due to the inhibition of mast cell synthesis of IL-4 and IL-13, which powerfully stimulate IgE generation. Even when already bound to omalizumab, IgE antibodies can still ligate allergens, thus trapping them and preventing their interactions with residual FcεRI-linked IgE anchored to mast cells [57]. Omalizumab cannot interact with FcεRI-bound IgE and, as a consequence, it does not induce mast cell/basophil degranulation, thus behaving mostly as a non-anaphylactogenic antibody. Given the peculiar mechanism of action of omalizumab

(Fig. 4.1), which competes with IgE receptors for binding to IgE-Cε3 domains, it is very important that this drug reaches a high molar excess, optimally characterized by an omalizumab/IgE ratio ranging from 7:1 to 15:1 [65]. Therefore, it is crucial that serum concentrations of IgE, as well as body weight, are taken into account when the individual dosages of omalizumab are established. If these rules are observed, after a single subcutaneous administration, omalizumab causes an 84–99 % reversible decrease in serum free IgE levels [66]. Firstly approved only for asthmatic patients exhibiting serum IgE concentrations ranging from 30 to 700 IU/mL, the use of omalizumab has been later extended in Europe to a maximum IgE level of 1,500 IU/mL [67, 68]. Omalizumab is characterized by a half-life of 19–22 days; following subcutaneous injection, this drug displays a bioavailability of 62 % and achieves its peak serum concentration within 7–8 days [69]. Due to these pharmacokinetic properties, omalizumab is usually administered subcutaneously every 4 weeks. Shorter intervals are chosen only for practical reasons when patients require relatively high drug doses. In fact, because the currently available vials of omalizumab contain 150 or 75 mg of drug, in order to avoid multiple subcutaneous injections at the same time, subjects needing more than 300 mg monthly are treated every 2 weeks.

Therapeutic Use of Omalizumab as Add-On Treatment for Asthma

Omalizumab binds circulating free IgE regardless of their antigen specificity, thereby being potentially useful for atopic asthma caused by either perennial or seasonal allergens, as well as by multiple sensitizations [70]. The initial clinical studies evaluating the efficacy of omalizumab in asthma showed that this anti-IgE antibody significantly inhibited early- and late-phase asthmatic reactions, triggered by inhaled allergens [71]. Subsequently, several randomized controlled trials have been undertaken in patients with moderate-to-severe asthma [72–77]. Overall, add-on treatment with omalizumab resulted to be very effective in reducing respiratory symptoms and especially asthma exacerbations, hospitalizations, emergency room visits and consumption of oral corticosteroids [8, 78, 79].

In particular, Busse et al., Solér et al. and Holgate et al. reported that omalizumab significantly decreased severe disease exacerbations in subjects with uncontrolled allergic asthma [72–74]. Moreover, Vignola et al. demonstrated that a 28-week add-on therapy course with omalizumab, performed in patients with moderate-to-severe asthma and concomitant rhinitis, markedly improved both Asthma Quality of Life Questionnaire (AQLQ) and Rhinitis Quality of Life Questionnaire (RQLQ) scores [75]; these results are very important because of the high relevance of allergic rhinitis as one of the most prevalent asthma comorbidities. Such findings have been further corroborated by a recent meta-analysis made by Tsabouri et al., referring to 11 trials carried out in inadequately controlled allergic rhinitic patients, which documented the remarkable efficacy of omalizumab in decreasing nasal symptom severity and daily rescue medication use [80]. A key study among those that evaluated omalizumab, named Investigation of Omalizumab in Severe Asthma Treatment (INNOVATE), was carried out by Humbert et al., who recruited 419 allergic subjects with uncontrolled severe asthma, characterized by recurrent disease exacerbations and marked bronchial obstruction (baseline $FEV_1 \geq 40-< 80\%$ predicted) [77]. When compared with the group treated with placebo, patients undergoing a 28-week add-on anti-IgE treatment with omalizumab experienced significant decreases in asthma exacerbations, emergency visits and requirements of oral corticosteroids. These results were also paralleled by relevant improvements in quality of life, asthma symptoms and peak expiratory flow (PEF) [77]. More recently, Hanania et al. enrolled 850 asthmatic patients with a wide age range (12–75 years), who underwent a comparative evaluation of omalizumab versus placebo after 48 weeks of add-on treatment; these authors found that omalizumab significantly lowered asthma symptoms and exacerbations and also reduced the daily need for short-acting rescue bronchodilators [81]. Another very interesting controlled trial involved a population of 419 subjects with moderate-to-severe persistent allergic asthma, including inner city children, adolescents and young adults, investigated by Busse et al. during 60 weeks of add-on treatment with omalizumab; these patients experienced a significant improvement in asthma control and an almost complete prevention of seasonal exacerbations, associated with a reduced intake of inhaled corticosteroids [82]. The efficacy of omalizumab in adults, adolescents and children with moderate-to-severe asthma has been also confirmed by a meta-analysis referring to eight selected placebo-controlled studies, published between 2001 and 2009 and globally involving more than 3,000 patients [83]. In particular, this systematic review considered as primary outcomes the reduction of asthma exacerbations and steroid utilization; secondary outcome measures included lung function, rescue medication use, asthma symptoms and health-related quality of life.

All these very convincing data, referring to placebo-controlled trials, have been further validated by an impressive number of real-life studies performed worldwide [84–93]. Besides confirming well-established outcomes including the decreases in annual rates of asthma exacerbations and hospitalizations, as well as the parallel improvements in quality of life, additional information has been gained by some of the most recent real-life investigations with regard to the relevance of comorbidities (chronic rhinosinusitis, nasal polyps, gastro-oesophageal reflux, obesity, aspirin intolerance) in the management of severe asthma. Indeed, by monitoring appropriate clinical and spirometric parameters like Asthma Control Test (ACT) score and forced expiratory volume in one second (FEV_1), as well as by measuring useful inflammatory biomarkers such as blood eosinophils and fractional exhaled nitric oxide (FeNO), Novelli et al. have shown that omalizumab provides a better control of severe asthma in patients without comorbidities [93]. This observation further emphasizes the role of omalizumab as a very precious adjunctive therapeutic tool, to be added within the context of an integrated treatment of severe allergic asthma that cannot absolutely disregard the necessity of adequately managing also concomitant diseases.

A key aspect regarding the management of severe asthma with omalizumab refers to the careful selection of candidate asthmatic subjects to treatment with this biologic drug. In our real-life experience, we usually obtain the best therapeutic results of add-on anti-IgE therapy in allergic asthma by treating severe, inadequately controlled and oral steroid-dependent asthmatics, experiencing very frequent disease exacerbations. In these patients, we have observed dramatic reductions in exacerbation rate and oral corticosteroid consumption, paralleled by remarkable changes in lung function (significant increases in both FEV_1 and FEV_1/FVC ratio) [94]. However, with regard to the effects of omalizumab on lung function, inconsistent data have been reported by various clinical trials [78]. Indeed, a decrease in free IgE does not necessarily affect FEV_1 and FEV_1/forced vital capacity (FVC) ratio [95]. Therefore, the effects of omalizumab on FEV_1 are quite controversial, and many studies have shown no significant change in such a functional parameter [78]. Nevertheless, some increases in FEV_1 have been occasionally recorded after several weeks of treatment with omalizumab [76, 96]. Furthermore, according to an open-label study carried out in patients with uncontrolled severe allergic asthma, randomized to receive best standard antiasthma therapy with or without omalizumab, in comparison with control values, a significant increase in percentage predicted FEV_1 has been observed throughout a 1-year period of anti-IgE treatment [97]. Moreover, a possible association can occur between the reduction of exacerbation frequency, elicited by omalizumab, and the recorded improvement of airflow limitation. This observation is consistent with the reported relationship between recurrence of asthma exacerbations and deterioration of lung function [98]. In particular, the exacerbation-prone phenotype of asthma may be characterized by a vicious pathogenetic circuit sustained by exacerbation-driven inflammation leading to bronchial narrowing, which in turn predisposes to repetitive exacerbation cycles. Such a self-perpetuating airway injury can thus be interrupted by omalizumab. Controversial findings have also been reported with regard to the effects of omalizumab on bronchial hyperresponsiveness. In fact, omalizumab does not seem to be able to affect the airway response to methacholine [99, 100]. However, bronchoconstrictive effectors that act directly on airway smooth muscle are not the most suitable stimuli in order to test the effects of omalizumab on bronchial hyperresponsiveness. Indeed, after 4 weeks of treatment, omalizumab significantly attenuated, in subjects with mild-to-moderate allergic asthma, the airway response to inhaled adenosine 5'-monophosphate (AMP) [100]. AMP-induced bronchoconstriction is due to stimulation of adenosine A_{2B} receptors located on mast cells; therefore, the bronchoprotection against AMP afforded by omalizumab is probably dependent on its capability of inhibiting mast cell activation synergistically triggered by allergens and other degranulating agents like AMP.

Very interesting are also the effects of omalizumab on various markers of airway inflammation. During the steroid reduction phase of a paediatric study performed in allergic asthmatic children, omalizumab was able to maintain FeNO at significantly lower levels with respect to placebo [101]. Moreover, omalizumab was also shown to be capable of decreasing eosinophil numbers in peripheral blood [102], as well as in induced sputum and bronchial biopsies [99]. This effect of omalizumab is likely due to the induction of eosinophil apoptosis. In particular, peripheral blood eosinophils are currently believed to be reliable inflammatory biomarkers, very useful to monitor the anti-inflammatory effects of omalizumab. In this regard, it is remarkable that a pooled analysis of data referring to several trials involving patients with moderate-to-severe persistent allergic asthma treated with omalizumab has found some degree of correlation between omalizumab-induced decrease in peripheral blood eosinophils and various clinical and functional outcomes; the latter included a reduced requirement for management of exacerbations with oral steroid bursts, an increased FEV_1 and a positive global evaluation of treatment effectiveness (GETE) by investigators [103]. Indeed, peripheral blood eosinophils can be considered as reliable biomarkers of Th2 cell-driven allergic inflammation, especially in association with high levels of FeNO and serum periostin. In this regard, the EXTRA study has demonstrated that high baseline values of these three biomarkers make it possible to predict a positive therapeutic response to omalizumab, expressed as a lower asthma exacerbation rate [104].

Anyway, the clinical responses to omalizumab treatment are variable and strictly individual. Currently, an overall physician's evaluation of omalizumab effects is suggested to be made after 16 weeks of therapy [105]. Basing their observations on GETE, Bousquet et al. found that patient responsiveness to omalizumab detected at the 16th week, persisted at the 32nd week [106]. However, among 71 allergic asthmatics who did not exhibit a clinical response within the first 16 weeks of treatment with omalizumab added to optimized asthma therapy, 27 subjects became omalizumab responders after further 16 weeks of treatment [106]. This report suggests that, by prolonging the initial observational time, it could be possible to extend the therapeutic benefits of omalizumab also to a subgroup of potential 'late responders', incorrectly classified as nonresponders on the basis of a 16-week period of clinical evaluation.

In addition to being really valuable in dampening allergic bronchial inflammation, omalizumab can also inhibit airway remodelling, which especially occurs in severe asthma (Fig. 4.2). Omalizumab might indeed interfere with the IgE-dependent synthetic activity of bronchial epithelium and airway smooth muscle cells, which remarkably contribute to the remodelling process. In fact, it has been reported that omalizumab was able to significantly decrease the production of TGF-β by bronchial epithelial cells, cultured in a medium containing atopic serum from a dust mite-sensitive patient and exposed to the stimulatory actions of IL-1β or ragweed allergen [107]. Through this mechanism, omalizumab could thus inhibit the fibrotic effects exerted by TGF-β in asthmatic airways. Furthermore, omalizumab significantly decreased the concentration of endothelin-1 (ET-1) in the exhaled breath condensate of patients with severe persistent allergic asthma [108]. ET-1 is a peptide mediator produced by vascular endothelial cells, bronchial epithelial cells and mast cells, which are actively involved in the pathogenesis of airway structural changes such as subepithelial fibrosis and proliferation of bronchial smooth muscle cells. The latter are also important targets of omalizumab, which can suppress their production of extracellular matrix proteins such as collagen [55]. The effects of anti-IgE treatment on airway remodelling have been shown through chest computed tomography (CT) scanning by Hoshino and Ohtawa, who after 16 weeks of add-on therapy with omalizumab detected a reduction of airway thickness associated with a concomitant enlargement of bronchial luminal area [109]. These imaging findings

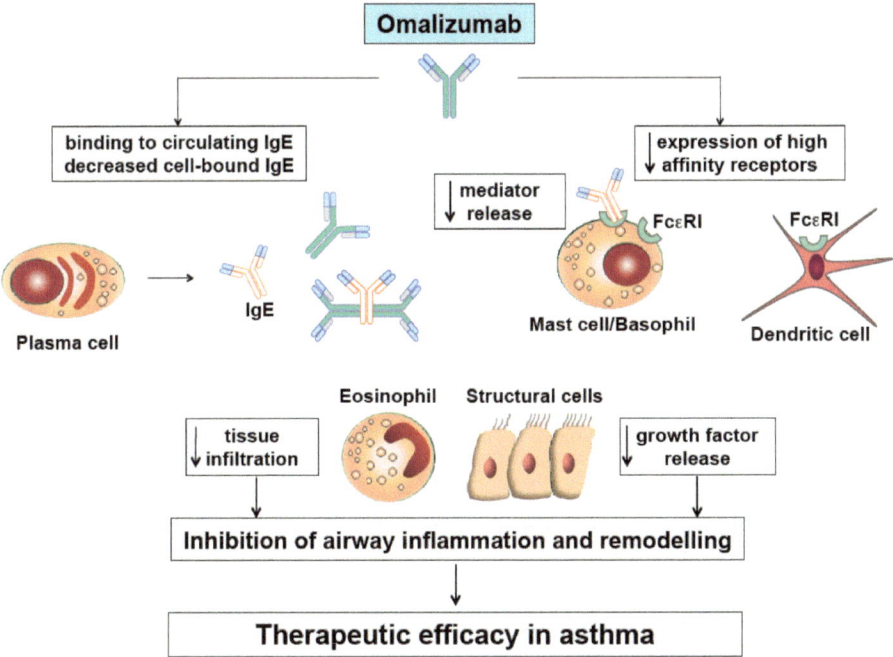

Fig. 4.2 Effects of omalizumab on airway inflammation and remodelling. Omalizumab-mediated inhibition of IgE binding to FcεRI expressed by immune-inflammatory cells results in a marked reduction of mediator release and eosinophilic allergic inflammation. IgE receptors are also present on structural cells such as bronchial epithelial cells and airway smooth muscle cells, whose IgE-dependent activity involved in airway remodelling could thus be effectively prevented by omalizumab (Reprinted from Ref. [8])

have been recently further confirmed by additional CT measurements made by Tajiri et al., who evidenced a significant decrease of bronchial wall thickness in adults with severe uncontrolled asthma, after 48 weeks of add-on treatment with omalizumab [110]. Such airway structural changes are likely related to a marked reduction in the thickness of epithelial reticular basement membrane (RBM), as demonstrated by Riccio et al. in bronchial biopsies taken from patients with severe allergic asthma before and after 12 months of anti-IgE therapy with omalizumab [111]. However, patient response evaluated in terms of changes in RBM thickness resulted to be very heterogeneous, thus identifying two distinct groups of responders and nonresponders to the anti-remodelling effects of omalizumab, respectively. This observation prompted the same research group to perform an elegant proteomic analysis of the bronchial biopsies obtained from both omalizumab responders and nonresponders [112]. The different protein profiles of these patients revealed an overexpression of galectin-3 in the airway tissues of responders, when compared to nonresponders. Therefore, galectin-3 can be probably considered as a potential and reliable biomarker capable of predicting the individual response to the inhibitory effect of omalizumab on bronchial remodelling.

Recent studies unexpectedly suggest that significant therapeutic benefits can also be achieved by patients with non-allergic asthma undergoing treatment with omalizumab. Indeed, de Llano et al. showed that a better asthma control was experienced by some non-atopic asthmatics after 2 years of add-on anti-IgE therapy [113]. Furthermore, a real-life study performed by Grimaldi-Bensouda et al. in a mixed group of patients including both allergic and non-allergic subjects with severe asthma showed that omalizumab remarkably lowered hospitalizations and emergency department visits; such positive outcomes were exhibited with similar patterns by allergic as well as non-allergic asthmatics [91]. Moreover, a placebo-controlled trial focusing on the evaluation of add-on omalizumab treatment in non-allergic patients with severe asthma was conducted by Garcia et al. [114]. These authors reported that, when compared to placebo, anti-IgE therapy with omalizumab decreased asthma exacerbation rate. In addition, a relevant FEV_1 increase and a significant reduction in FcεRI expression on basophils and plasmacytoid dendritic cells (pDC) were also recorded [114]. These favourable results, obtained in patients with non-allergic asthma receiving omalizumab, might be explained by at least two plausible arguments [115]. Accordingly to a first hypothesis, asthmatic patients defined as non-allergic on the basis of negative skin prick tests associated with the absence of allergen-specific serum IgE antibodies could instead be truly atopic. In particular, they might be sensitized to undefined allergens, within the context of a local immune response occurring inside the airways, without any systemic spillover. Another explanation could be based on a predominant effect of omalizumab at level of pDC, which also in non-atopic subjects plays a key physiologic role in innate immunity, especially targeted against viral infections. FcεRI-bound IgE impair such an antiviral function of pDC, which can thus be restored by omalizumab through inhibition of FcεRI activation, as well as via downregulation of pDC FcεRI expression. By means of these mechanisms, omalizumab could thereby exert an effective protection against asthma exacerbations, which are often triggered by respiratory viruses in both allergic and non-allergic patients [115].

In clinical practice, a crucial issue related to the use of omalizumab regards the duration of anti-IgE treatment. The mechanism of action of omalizumab, based on competitive binding to the Cε3 domain of the constant fragment of IgE, would suggest that this drug should be used according to a life-long schedule in order to block IgE functions. Indeed, interruption of a long-term add-on therapy with omalizumab can be followed within a few months by a relapse in asthma symptoms and exacerbations, possibly associated with an increased intensity of allergen-induced reactions assessed by skin prick test [116, 117]. However, a small-size investigation carried out by Nopp et al. demonstrated that after a 6-year treatment with omalizumab, discontinuation of anti-IgE therapy was associated, in 12 out of 18 enrolled patients, with a persistence for at least 3 years of the achieved improvements in asthma symptoms and lung function [118]. This report is consistent with more recent data, recorded by Baena-Cagnani et al. in some Argentinian asthmatic children, who remained completely free of respiratory symptoms during the first 3 years of follow-up after omalizumab withdrawal [119]. These authors thus speculate that anti-IgE therapy could modify the natural history of moderate-to-severe uncontrolled asthma, and this potential effect might mainly be due to a modulatory action of omalizumab on bronchial remodelling. On the contrary, in 9 out of 11 Polish adult asthmatic patients forced to stop anti-IgE treatment because of a change in reimbursement rules, Kuprys-Lipinska and Kuna noticed a recurrence of severe asthma exacerbations within the first 5 months since interruption of treatment with omalizumab [120]. Such a negative outcome was also associated with worsened asthma control and quality of life, evaluated by Asthma Control Questionnaire (ACQ) and AQLQ, respectively. These apparent discrepancies can perhaps be explained by the different age of the asthmatic patients enrolled in the latter two studies. Indeed, the development of the natural course of asthma might be more susceptible to omalizumab-induced changes at earlier stages during childhood, rather than later in life. Anyway, given the currently available limited information, more studies are needed to further explore the possible effects of omalizumab on the pathobiologic evolution of asthma. Hence, in consideration of the individual susceptibility to an eventual cessation of anti-IgE treatment, careful prudence should be shared by both clinicians and patients in taking decisions regarding a possible stop of omalizumab administration after several years of treatment [121], especially in adult asthmatics. In this regard, the best choice should probably be made by carefully deciding on a case-by-case basis.

Safety and Tolerability Profile of Omalizumab

Omalizumab is usually very well tolerated. Indeed, the most reported side effects are represented by local and limited reactions occurring at injection sites. Sometimes, omalizumab-treated patients can also experience nausea, headache or tiredness. Overall, add-on therapy with omalizumab is characterized by a pattern of adverse events which is very similar to that observed during treatment with placebo [122]. Even if omalizumab is a non-anaphylactogenic antibody, anaphylactic and anaphylactoid reactions have been occasionally reported. However, their occurrence is very rare, being characterized by a 0.09 % rate among omalizumab-treated patients [123]. Moreover, anti-omalizumab antibodies are not detectable in omalizumab-treated patients. Initial studies had raised a major concern, referring to a slight increase in the cases of cancer among patients receiving omalizumab, as compared with placebo-treated subjects [66]. Nevertheless, no difference in the incidence of malignancies has been detected between patients undergoing omalizumab treatment and the general population [124, 125]. Isolated reports of Churg-Strauss syndrome, possibly occurring during add-on therapy with omalizumab, have been published [126–128]. However, it is still debated if there is a clear causal relationship between omalizumab treatment and Churg-Strauss syndrome, or rather if this disease could be pre-existing and then unmasked by the progressive reduction and subsequent suspension of systemic corticosteroid therapy. Conversely, omalizumab has also been considered as a potential treatment for Churg-Strauss syndrome [129]. Though IgE antibodies are involved in immune defence against parasitic infections, the risk of developing such infestations appears to be very low during treatment with omalizumab [130]. Indeed, evolutionary theories suggest that although IgE are very important in protecting animals and even humans living in primitive habitats, these antibodies seem to have become nonessential in many regions of the world characterized by relatively clean house and community environments. However, because of some reports referring to a slight increase in helminthic infections associated with omalizumab use [130], patients living in or travelling to areas where these parasitic infestations are endemic should be advised about such a potential risk. The cardiovascular safety profile of omalizumab seems to be well documented by an accurate review of eight controlled studies collectively involving more than 3,000 patients, who exhibited an omalizumab-related cardiovascular risk not significantly different from that occurring in placebo-treated groups [83]. With respect to controls, no risk of spontaneous abortion has been found in small-size populations of pregnant women receiving omalizumab during their pregnancy [131]. Furthermore, no apparent increases in the prevalence of major anomalies have been recently reported in children born from omalizumab-treated mothers [132]. On the basis of the above considerations and according to the opinions of both clinicians and patients, omalizumab is currently and widely believed to be very safe. However, similarly to all monoclonal antibodies used as biologic therapies, a continuous and careful monitoring is necessary, especially because the numbers of omalizumab-treated patients are progressively increasing worldwide [133].

Cost-Effectiveness of Omalizumab Treatment for Severe Asthma

Although omalizumab treatment seems to be highly expensive, however this biological therapy can be cost-effective if it is restricted to selected patients with severe persistent and uncontrolled asthma, who respond within 16 weeks with a marked improvement in disease control [78, 134]. This perception, inferred from medical practice, has been confirmed by detailed assessments of the incremental cost-effectiveness ratio (ICER) of adding omalizumab to standard therapy [135], based on data obtained from the real-life, 1-year randomized open-label ETOPA study [76]. To determine the ICER for omalizumab, the cost/quality-adjusted life years (QALY) ratio was calculated. In particular, Canada was used as reference country, and only subjects receiving high doses of inhaled corticosteroids plus long-acting β_2-adrenoceptor agonists were considered. Based on such reliable criteria, the authors of this analysis concluded that 'omalizumab add-on therapy in patients with severe persistent asthma results in a cost-per-QALY ratio that compares favourably with other uses of scarce healthcare resources that are recommended by national reimbursement bodies and could be considered cost-effective' [135]. Positive evaluations in terms of cost-effectiveness of omalizumab treatment have also been performed in other countries such as the USA, Sweden, the Netherlands and Italy [136–140]. The cost-saving effects of omalizumab depend on relevant decreases in both direct and indirect costs due to asthma. Direct costs, which also include further expenses for additional drugs used to manage worsening symptoms, are primarily related to asthma exacerbations requiring hospitalization or access to emergency department or leading to unscheduled visits made by general practitioners or pulmonologists. Indirect costs refer to the enhanced social burden arising from the loss of school and working days, possibly causing significant reductions of work productivity and employment rates.

Overall, comparative economic assessments of the cost-effectiveness of omalizumab have confirmed that, in patients with severe persistent allergic asthma, add-on therapy is comparable to or more favourable than other biologic treatments for chronic disorders such as rheumatoid arthritis, Crohn's disease and multiple sclerosis [141]. This economically advantageous utilization of omalizumab is thus linked to its sparing effect on the very high percentage of the global asthma budget consumed by the patient groups suffering from the most severe disease forms.

Future Perspectives of Anti-IgE Therapy

The therapeutic success of omalizumab in asthma treatment has prompted the development of further anti-IgE antibodies. In particular, ligelizumab is a humanized IgG1 monoclonal antibody which binds with a 50-fold higher in vitro affinity than omalizumab to the Cε3 domain of IgE [142, 143]. This higher in vitro affinity translated into a six- to ninefold greater potency in vivo [142]. Two placebo-controlled clinical trials were performed in atopic patients, both including an open-label omalizumab arm; in the first trial, ligelizumab was administered as single intravenous doses ranging from 0.1 to 10 mg/kg, whereas in the second study, two to four subcutaneous drug doses of 0.2–4 mg/kg were administered at 2-week intervals [142]. In comparison to omalizumab, ligelizumab induced a greater and longer reduction of free serum IgE, as well as of IgE expressed on the surface of circulating basophils. Ligelizumab was also more effective than omalizumab in inhibiting skin prick test responses to allergens. With regard to safety and tolerability, intravenous ligelizumab caused mild-to-moderate urticaria in 4 of the 60 subjects who completed the intravenous study. With regard to the other mild-to-moderate adverse events reported during both trials, mainly including headache and upper respiratory infections, only the local reactions occurring at injection sites appeared to be related to study drug. Therefore, given its remarkable potency of action, ligelizumab could be potentially used also by allergic asthmatic patients not eligible for treatment with omalizumab because of their excessive serum IgE levels.

More recently, a new anti-IgE antibody (MEDI4212) was developed, which is characterized by a dual mechanism of action, simultaneously inhibiting both synthesis and effects of IgE [144]. Indeed, MEDI4212 is able not only to bind with high-affinity soluble IgE but also to deplete IgE-producing B cells. With respect to the parental IgE-binding antibody, MEDI4212 was generated by changing the sugar content through the removal of a fucose moiety (afucosylation) in the oligo-saccharide located between the two Fc arms. This structural change resulted in a remarkably higher affinity of MEDI4212 for the FcγRIIIa receptor present on the surface of effector cells such as natural killer (NK) cells and monocytes/macrophages. In addition to linking human IgE expressed on B-cell membrane via its Fab fragments, this new antibody was thus shown to be also capable of interacting through the Fc portion with FcγRIIIa-bearing effector cells. Such a strong dual interaction promoted a process of antibody-dependent cellular cytotoxicity (ADCC), resulting in apoptosis mediated by effector cells via release of perforin and granzyme B. This complex mechanism can cause the elimination of B lymphocytes carrying membrane-bound IgE and the consequent depletion of IgE-secreting plasma cells. Similarly to omalizumab, MEDI4212 is able to induce rapid decreases in circulating free IgE, but in addition it can also elicit a long-term reduction of IgE synthesis. Indeed, the premature death of IgE expressing memory B lymphocytes prevents their differentiation in IgE-secreting plasma cells. MEDI4212 may thereby interfere very effectively with two crucial events of the allergic cascade, including the upstream production of IgE and the downstream linkage of IgE to FcεRI receptors expressed by mast cells, basophils and dendritic cells. Hence, a dual IgE neutralizing and lowering antibody could widen the treatable population of severe allergic asthmatics, thereby also including patients with very high IgE levels.

Concluding Remarks

The introduction of omalizumab in clinical practice represented a very important advance towards a better management of severe uncontrolled asthma. Omalizumab has been the first and for a long time the unique biologic drug registered for asthma therapy, making it possible to remarkably improve, when added to standard anti-asthma treatment, respiratory symptoms, quality of life and especially exacerbation rate [78]. Both placebo-controlled studies and real-life trials have unequivocally demonstrated the therapeutic effectiveness of omalizumab, due to its capability of markedly blunting allergic bronchial inflammation. These positive pharmacologic features are also associated with a very good profile of safety and tolerability. Moreover, current experimental evidence suggests that omalizumab can also interfere with the cellular and molecular mechanisms underlying airway remodelling, thus possibly behaving as a disease-modifying agent, in addition to being an effective anti-inflammatory drug (Fig. 4.2). Finally, recent studies seem to indicate that the therapeutic use of omalizumab could potentially be extended to some patients with non-atopic severe asthma. Of course, these new findings could widen the eligibility of asthmatic subjects for add-on anti-IgE treatment, but such enlarged applications of omalizumab will undoubtedly require an accurate search for reliable asthma biomarkers, in order to reasonably predict the potential success of this biologic drug according to a personalized therapeutic approach. Moreover, the latest molecular developments leading to the generation of new anti-IgE antibodies can potentially provide a further step forward in the modern treatment of atopic diseases.

References

1. Froidure A, Mouthuy J, Durham SR, et al. Asthma phenotypes and IgE responses. Eur Respir J. 2016;47:304–19.
2. Gould HJ, Sutton BJ. IgE in allergy and asthma today. Nat Rev Immunol. 2008;8:205–17.
3. Hentges F, Leonard C, Arumugam K, et al. Immune responses to inhalant mammalian allergens. Front Immunol. 2014;5:234.
4. Dullaers M, De Bruyne R, Ramadani F, et al. The who, where and when of IgE in allergic airway disease. J Allergy Clin Immunol. 2012;129:635–45.
5. Ishizaka K, Ishizaka T. Identification of γE antibodies as a carrier of reaginic activity. J Immunol. 1967;6:1187–98.
6. Pelaia G, Vatrella A, Calabrese C, et al. New perspectives in asthma treatment. Allergy. 2000;55 suppl 61:60–6.
7. Global strategy for asthma management and prevention. Global Initiative for Asthma (GINA). 2016. Available from: http://www.ginasthma.org/.
8. Pelaia G, Vatrella A, Busceti MT, et al. Anti-IgE therapy with omalizumab for severe asthma: current concepts and potential developments. Curr Drug Targets. 2015;16:171–8.
9. Takhar P, Corrigan CJ, Smurthwaite L, et al. Class switch recombination to IgE in the bronchial mucosa of atopic and nonatopic patients with asthma. J Allergy Clin Immunol. 2007;119:213–8.
10. Altin J, Shen C, Liston A. Understanding the genetic regulation of IgE production. Blood Rev. 2010;24:163–9.
11. Campbell AM, Vachier I, Chanez P, et al. Expression of the high-affinity receptor for IgE on bronchial epithelial cells of asthmatics. Am J Respir Cell Mol Biol. 1998;19:92–7.
12. Gounni AS, Wellemans V, Yang J, et al. Human airway smooth muscle cells express the high affinity receptor for IgE (FcεRI): a critical role of FcεRI in human airway smooth muscle cell function. J Immunol. 2005;175:2613–21.
13. Wan T, Beavil RL, Fabiane SM, et al. The crystal structure of IgE Fc reveals an asymmetrically bent conformation. Nat Immunol. 2002;3:681–6.
14. Cao L, Yu K, Banh C, et al. Quantitative time-resolved phosphoproteomic analysis of mast cell signaling. J Immunol. 2007;179:5864–76.
15. Saitoh S, Arudchandran R, Manetz TS, et al. LAT is essential for FcεRI-mediated mast cell activation. Immunity. 2000;12:525–35.
16. Gilfillan AM, Tkaczyk C. Integrated signalling pathways for mast-cell activation. Nat Rev Immunol. 2006;6:218–30.
17. Holgate ST. Pathogenesis of asthma. Clin Exp Allergy. 2008;38:872–97.
18. Cruse G, Kaur D, Yang W, et al. Activation of human lung mast cells by monomeric immunoglobulin E. Eur Respir J. 2005;25:858–63.
19. Cruse G, Cockerill S, Bradding P. IgE alone promotes human lung mast cell survival through the autocrine production of IL-6. BMC Immunol. 2008;9:2.
20. Matsuda K, Piliponsky AM, Iikura M, et al. Monomeric IgE enhances human mast cell chemokine production: IL-4 augments and dexamethasone suppresses the response. J Allergy Clin Immunol. 2005;116:1357–63.
21. Hibbert RG, Teriete P, Grundy GJ, et al. The structure of human CD23 and its interactions with IgE and CD21. J Exp Med. 2005;202:751–60.
22. Acharya M, Borland G, Edkins AL, et al. CD23/FcεRII: molecular multi-tasking. Clin Exp Immunol. 2010;162:12–23.
23. Campbell AM, Vignola AM, Chanez P, et al. Low-affinity receptor for IgE on human bronchial epithelial cells in asthma. Immunology. 1994;82:506–8.
24. Lantz CS, Yamaguchi M, Oettgen HC, et al. IgE regulates mouse basophil FcεRI expression in vivo. J Immunol. 1997;158:2517–21.
25. Yamaguchi M, Lantz CS, Oettgen HC, et al. IgE enhances mouse mast cell FcεRI expression in vitro and in vivo: evidence for a novel amplification mechanism in IgE-dependent reactions. J Exp Med. 1997;17:663–72.

26. Kisselgof AB, Oettgen HC. The expression of murine B cell CD23, in vivo, is regulated by its ligand IgE. Int Immunol. 1998;10:1377–84.
27. Saini SS, Klion AD, Holland SM, et al. The relationship between serum IgE and surface levels of FcεR on human leukocytes in various diseases: correlation of expression with FcεRI on basophils but not on monocytes or eosinophils. J Allergy Clin Immunol. 2000;106:514–20.
28. Borkowski TA, Jouvin MH, Lin SY, et al. Minimal requirements for IgE-mediated regulation of surface FcεRI. J Immunol. 2001;167:1290–6.
29. Kalesnikoff J, Huber M, Lam V, et al. Monomeric IgE stimulates signaling pathways in mast cells that lead to cytokine production and cell survival. Immunity. 2001;14:801–11.
30. Sihra BS, Kon OM, Grant JA, et al. Expression of high-affinity IgE receptors (FcεRI) on peripheral blood basophils, monocytes, and eosinophils in atopic and nonatopic subjects: relationship to total serum IgE concentrations. J Allergy Clin Immunol. 1997;99:699–706.
31. Foster B, Metcalfe DD, Prussin C. Human dendritic cell 1 and dendritic cell 2 subsets express FcεRI: correlation with serum IgE and allergic asthma. J Allergy Clin Immunol. 2003;112:1132–8.
32. MacGlashan Jr D. IgE receptor and signal transduction in mast cells and basophils. Curr Opin Immunol. 2008;20:717–23.
33. Weskamp G, Ford JW, Sturgill J, et al. ADAM10 is a principal 'sheddase' of the low-affinity immunoglobulin E receptor CD23. Nat Immunol. 2006;12:1293–8.
34. Platzer B, Ruiter F, van der Mee J, et al. Soluble IgE receptors elements of the IgE network. Immunol Lett. 2011;141:36–44.
35. Kraft S, Kinet J-P. New developments in FcεRI regulation, function and inhibition. Nat Rev Immunol. 2007;7:365–78.
36. Dehlink E, Platzer B, Baker AH, et al. A soluble form of the high affinity IgE receptor, FcεRI, circulates in human serum. PLoS One. 2011;6:e19098.
37. Lee BW, Simmons Jr CF, Wileman T, et al. Intracellular cleavage of newly synthesized low affinity Fcε receptor (FcεR2) provides a second pathway for the generation of the 28-kDa soluble FcεR2 fragment. J Immunol. 1989;142:1614–20.
38. Mathews JA, Gibb DR, Chen BH, et al. CD23 disintegrin and metalloproteinase 10 (ADAM10) is also required for CD23 sorting into B cell-derived exosomes. J Biol Chem. 2010;285:37531–41.
39. McCloskey N, Hunt J, Beavil RL, et al. Soluble CD23 monomers inhibit and oligomers stimulate IgE synthesis in human B cells. J Biol Chem. 2007;282:24083–91.
40. MacKinnon AC, Farnworth SL, Hodkinson PS, et al. Regulation of alternative macrophage activation by galectin-3. J Immunol. 2008;180:2650–8.
41. Dumic J, Dabelic S, Flögel M. Galectin-3: an open-ended story. Biochim Biophys Acta. 2006;1760:616–35.
42. Liu FT. Regulatory roles of galectins in the immune response. Int Arch Allergy Immunol. 2005;136:385–400.
43. Liu FT, Rabinovich GA. Galectins: regulators of acute and chronic inflammation. Ann N Y Acad Sci. 2010;1183:158–82.
44. Maurer D, Fiebiger S, Ebner C, et al. Peripheral blood dendritic cells express FcεRI as a complex composed of FcεRI α- FcεRI γ-chains and can use this receptor for IgE-mediated allergen presentation. J Immunol. 1996;157:607–16.
45. Maurer D, Fiebiger E, Reininger B, et al. FcεRI on dendritic cells delivers IgE-bound multivalent antigens into a cathepsin S-dependent pathway of MHC class II presentation. J Immunol. 1998;161:2731–9.
46. Khan SH, Grayson MH. Cross-linking IgE augments human conventional dendritic cell production of CC chemokine ligand 28. J Allergy Clin Immunol. 2010;125:265–7.
47. Lynch JP, Mazzone SB, Rogers MJ, et al. The plasmacytoid dendritic cell: at the cross-roads in asthma. Eur Respir J. 2014;43:264–75.
48. Soussi Gounni A, Lamkhioued B, Ochiai K, Tanaka Y, Delaporte E, et al. High-affinity IgE receptor on eosinophils is involved in defence against parasites. Nature. 1994;367:183–6.

49. Rajakulasingam K, Durham SR, O'Brien F, et al. Enhanced expression of high-affinity IgE receptor (FcεRI) α chain in human allergen-induced rhinitis with co-localization to mast cells, macrophages, eosinophils, and dendritic cells. J Allergy Clin Immunol. 1997;100:78–86.
50. Smith SJ, Ying S, Meng Q, et al. Blood eosinophils from atopic donors express messenger RNA for the α, β, and γ subunits of the high-affinity IgE receptor (FcεRI) and intracellular, but not cell surface, subunit protein. J Allergy Clin Immunol. 2000;105:309–17.
51. Kim IS, Kim MJ, Kim DH, et al. Different anti-apoptotic effects of normal and asthmatic serum on normal eosinophil apoptosis depending on house dust mite-specific IgE. Mol Biol Rep. 2013;40:5875–81.
52. Palaniyandi S, Tomei E, Li Z, et al. CD23-dependent transcytosis of IgE and immune complex across the polarized human respiratory epithelial cells. J Immunol. 2011;186:3484–96.
53. Palaniyandi S, Liu X, Periasamy S, et al. Inhibition of CD23-mediated IgE transcytosis suppresses the initiation and development of allergic airway inflammation. Mucosal Immunol. 2015;8:1262–74.
54. Redhu NS, Gounni AS. The high affinity IgE receptor (FcεRI) expression and function in airway smooth muscle. Pulm Pharmacol Ther. 2013;26:86–94.
55. Roth M, Zhong J, Zumkeller C, et al. The role of IgE-receptors in IgE-dependent airway smooth muscle cell remodelling. PLoS One. 2013;8:e56015.
56. Presta LG, Lahr SJ, Shields RL, et al. Humanization of an antibody directed against IgE. J Immunol. 1993;151:2623–32.
57. Spector S. Omalizumab efficacy in allergic disease. Panminerva Med. 2004;46:141–8.
58. Hochhaus G, Brookman L, Fox H, et al. Pharmacodynamics of omalizumab: implications for optimised dosing strategy and clinical efficacy in the treatment of allergic asthma. Curr Med Res Opin. 2003;19:491–8.
59. Fox JA, Hotaling TE, Struble C, et al. Tissue distribution and complex generation with IgE of an anti-IgE antibody after intravenous administration in cynomolgus monkeys. J Pharmacol Exp Ther. 1996;279:1000–8.
60. Chang TW, Wu PC, Hsu CL, et al. Anti-IgE antibodies for the treatment of IgE-mediated allergic diseases. Adv Immunol. 2007;93:63–119.
61. Presta L, Shields R, O' Connell L, et al. The binding site of a human immunoglobulin E for its high affinity receptor. J Biol Chem. 1994;269:26368–73.
62. Domingo C. Omalizumab for severe asthma: efficacy beyond the atopic patient? Drugs. 2014;74:521–33.
63. Noga O, Hanf G, Brachmann I, et al. Effect of omalizumab treatment on peripheral eosinophil and T-lymphocyte function in patients with allergic asthma. J Allergy Clin Immunol. 2006;117:1493–9.
64. Holgate S, Casale T, Wenzel S, et al. The anti-inflammatory effects of omalizumab confirm the central role of IgE in allergic inflammation. J Allergy Clin Immunol. 2005;115:459–65.
65. Marcus P. Incorporating anti-IgE (omalizumab) therapy in clinical practice: practice management implications. Chest. 2006;129:466–74.
66. Miller CWT, Krishnaswamy N, Johnston C, et al. Severe asthma and the omalizumab option. Clin Mol Allergy. 2008;6:4.
67. Domingo C, Pacheco A, Hinojosa M, et al. The relevance of IgE in the pathogenesis of allergy: the effect of an anti-IgE drug in asthma and other diseases. Recent Pat Inflamm Allergy Drug Discov. 2007;1:151–64.
68. Buhl R, Marco AG, Cohen D, et al. Eligibility for treatment with omalizumab in Italy and Germany. Respir Med. 2014;108:50–6.
69. Hendeles L, Sorkness CA. Anti-immunoglobulin E therapy with omalizumab for asthma. Ann Pharmacother. 2007;41:1397–410.
70. D'Amato G. Role of anti-IgE monoclonal antibody (omalizumab) in the treatment of bronchial asthma and allergic respiratory diseases. Eur J Pharmacol. 2006;533:302–7.
71. Fahy JV, Fleming HE, Wong HH, et al. The effect of an anti-IgE monoclonal antibody on the early- and late-phase responses to allergen inhalation in asthmatic subjects. Am J Respir Crit Care Med. 1997;155:1828–34.

72. Busse W, Corren J, Lanier BQ, et al. Omalizumab, anti-IgE recombinant humanized mono-
    clonal antibody for the treatment of severe allergic asthma. J Allergy Clin Immunol.
    2001;108:184–90.
73. Solèr M, Matz J, Townley R, et al. The anti-IgE antibody omalizumab reduces exacerbations
    and steroid requirement in allergic asthmatics. Eur Respir J. 2001;18:254–61.
74. Holgate ST, Chuchalin AG, Hebert J, et al. Efficacy and tolerability of a recombinant anti-
    immunoglobulin E antibody (omalizumab) in severe allergic asthma. Clin Exp Allergy.
    2004;34:632–8.
75. Vignola AM, Humbert M, Bousquet J, et al. Efficacy and tolerability of anti-immunoglobulin
    E therapy with omalizumab in patients with concomitant allergic asthma and persistent aller-
    gic rhinitis: SOLAR. Allergy. 2004;59:709–17.
76. Ayres JG, Higgins B, Chilvers ER, et al. Efficacy and tolerability of anti-immunoglobulin E
    therapy with omalizumab in patients with poorly controlled (moderate-to-severe) allergic
    asthma. Allergy. 2004;59:701–8.
77. Humbert M, Beasley R, Ayres J, et al. Benefits of omalizumab as add-on therapy in patients
    with severe persistent asthma who are inadequately controlled despite best available therapy
    (GINA 2002 step 4 treatment): INNOVATE. Allergy. 2005;60:309–16.
78. Price D. The use of omalizumab in asthma. Prim Care Respir J. 2008;17:62–72.
79. Pelaia G, Vatrella A, Maselli R. The potential of biologics for the treatment of asthma. Nat
    Rev Drug Discov. 2012;11:958–72.
80. Tsabouri S, Tseretopoulou X, Priftis K, et al. Omalizumab for the treatment of inadequately
    controlled allergic rhinitis: a systematic review and meta-analysis of randomized clinical tri-
    als. J Allergy Clin Immunol Pract. 2014;2:332–40.
81. Hanania NA, Alpan O, Hamilos DL, et al. Omalizumab in severe allergic asthma inadequately
    controlled with standard therapy: a randomized trial. Ann Intern Med. 2011;154:573–82.
82. Busse WW, Morgan WJ, Gergen PJ, et al. Randomized trial of omalizumab (anti-IgE) for
    asthma in inner-city children. N Engl J Med. 2011;364:1005–15.
83. Rodrigo GJ, Neffen H, Castro-Rodriguez JA. Efficacy and safety of subcutaneous omali-
    zumab vs placebo as add-on therapy to corticosteroids for children and adults with asthma: a
    systematic review. Chest. 2011;139:28–35.
84. Molimard M, de Blay F, Didier A, et al. Effectiveness of omalizumab (Xolair) in the first
    patients treated in real-life practice in France. Respir Med. 2008;102:71–6.
85. Korn S, Thielen A, Seyfried S, et al. Omalizumab in patients with severe persistent allergic
    asthma in a real-life setting in Germany. Respir Med. 2009;103:1725–31.
86. Brusselle G, Michils A, Louis R, et al. Real-life effectiveness of omalizumab in patients with
    severe persistent allergic asthma: The PERSIST study. Respir Med. 2009;103:1633–42.
87. Cazzola M, Camiciottoli G, Bonavia M, et al. Italian real-life experience of omalizumab.
    Respir Med. 2010;104:1410–6.
88. Molimard M, Buhl R, Niven R, et al. Omalizumab reduces oral corticosteroid use in patients
    with severe allergic asthma: real-life data. Respir Med. 2010;104:1381–5.
89. Storms W, Bowdish MS, Farrar JR. Omalizumab and asthma control in patients with
    moderate-to-severe allergic asthma: a 6-year pragmatic data review. Allergy Asthma Proc.
    2012;33:172–7.
90. Tzortzaki EG, Georgiou A, Kampas D, et al. Long-term omalizumab treatment in severe
    allergic asthma: the South-Eastern Mediterranean "real-life" experience. Pulm Pharmacol
    Ther. 2012;25:77–82.
91. Grimaldi-Bensouda L, Zureik M, Aubier M, et al. Does omalizumab make a difference to the
    real-life treatment of asthma exacerbations? Results from a large cohort of patients with
    severe uncontrolled asthma. Chest. 2013;143:398–405.
92. Lopez Tiro JJ, Contreras EA, Del Pozo ME, et al. Real life study of three years omalizumab
    in patients with difficult-to-control asthma. Allergol Immunopathol. 2015;43:120–6.
93. Novelli F, Latorre M, Vergura L, et al. Asthma control in severe asthmatics under treatment
    with omalizumab: a cross-sectional observational study in Italy. Pulm Pharmacol Ther.
    2015;31:123–9.

94. Pelaia G, Gallelli L, Romeo P, et al. Omalizumab decreases exacerbation frequency, oral intake of corticosteroids and peripheral blood eosinophils in atopic patients with uncontrolled asthma. Int J Clin Pharmacol Ther. 2011;49:713–21.
95. Ledford DK. Omalizumab: overview of pharmacology and efficacy in asthma. Expert Opin Biol Ther. 2009;9:933–43.
96. Lanier BQ, Corren J, Lumry W, et al. Omalizumab is effective in the long-term control of severe allergic asthma. Ann Allergy Asthma Immunol. 2003;91:154–9.
97. Holgate S, Smith N, Massanari M, et al. Effects of omalizumab on markers of inflammation in patients with allergic asthma. Allergy. 2009;64:1728–36.
98. Bai TR, Vonk JM, Postma DS, et al. Severe exacerbations predict excess lung function decline in asthma. Eur Respir J. 2007;30:452–6.
99. Djukanovic R, Wilson SJ, Kraft M, et al. Effects of treatment with anti-immunoglobulin E antibody omalizumab on airway inflammation in allergic asthma. Am J Respir Crit Care Med. 2004;170:583–93.
100. Prieto L, Gutiérrez V, Colas C, et al. Effect of omalizumab on adenosine 5'-monophosphate responsiveness in subjects with allergic asthma. Int Arch Allergy Immunol. 2006;139: 122–31.
101. Silkoff PE, Romero FA, Gupta N, et al. Exhaled nitric oxide in children with asthma receiving Xolair (omalizumab), a monoclonal anti-immunoglobulin E antibody. Pediatrics. 2004;113:e308–12.
102. Noga O, Hanf G, Kunkel G. Immunological and clinical changes in allergic asthmatics following treatment with omalizumab. Int Arch Allergy Immunol. 2003;131:46–52.
103. Massanari M, Holgate ST, Busse WW, et al. Effect of omalizumab on peripheral blood eosinophilia in allergic asthma. Respir Med. 2010;104:188–96.
104. Hanania NA, Wenzel S, Rosén K, et al. Exploring the effects of omalizumab in allergic asthma: an analysis of biomarkers in the EXTRA study. Am J Respir Crit Care Med. 2013;187:804–11.
105. Bousquet J, Rabe K, Humbert M, et al. Predicting and evaluating response to omalizumab in patients with severe allergic asthma. Respir Med. 2007;101:1483–92.
106. Bousquet J, Siergiejko Z, Swiebocka E, et al. Persistency of response to omalizumab therapy in severe allergic (IgE-mediated) asthma. Allergy. 2011;66:671–8.
107. Huang YC, Leyko B, Frier M. Effects of omalizumab and budesonide on markers of inflammation in human bronchial epithelial cells. Ann Allergy Asthma Immunol. 2005;95:443–51.
108. Zietkowski Z, Skiepko R, Tomasiak-Lozowska MM, et al. Anti-IgE therapy with omalizumab decreases endothelin-1 in exhaled breath condensate of patients with severe persistent allergic asthma. Respiration. 2010;80:534–42.
109. Hoshino M, Ohtawa J. Effects of adding omalizumab, an anti-immunoglobulin E antibody, on airway wall thickening in asthma. Respiration. 2012;83:520–8.
110. Tajiri T, Niimi A, Matsumoto H, et al. Comprehensive efficacy of omalizumab for severe refractory asthma: a time-series observational study. Ann Allergy Asthma Immunol. 2014; 113:470–5.
111. Riccio AM, Dal Negro RW, Micheletto C, et al. Omalizumab modulates bronchial reticular basement membrane thickness and eosinophil infiltration in severe persistent allergic asthma patients. Int J Immunopathol Pharmacol. 2012;25:475–84.
112. Mauri P, Riccio AM, Rossi R, et al. Proteomics of bronchial biopsies: galectin-3 as a predictive biomarker of airway remodelling modulation in omalizumab-treated severe asthma patients. Immunol Lett. 2014;162:2–10.
113. de Llano LP, Vennera Mdel C, Alvarez FJ, et al. Effects of omalizumab in non-atopic asthma: results from a Spanish multicenter registry. J Asthma. 2013;50:296–301.
114. Garcia G, Magnan A, Chiron R, et al. A proof of concept randomized-controlled trial of omalizumab in patients with severe difficult to control nonatopic asthma. Chest. 2013;144:411–9.
115. Lommatzsch M, Korn S, Buhl R, et al. Against all odds: anti-IgE for intrinsic asthma? Thorax. 2014;69:94–6.

116. Pelaia G, Gallelli L, Renda T, et al. Update on optimal use of omalizumab in management of asthma. J Asthma Allergy. 2011;4:49–59.
117. Corren J, Shapiro G, Reimann J, et al. Allergen skin tests and free IgE levels during reduction and cessation of omalizumab therapy. J Allergy Clin Immunol. 2008;121:506–11.
118. Nopp A, Johansson SG, Adédoyin J, et al. After 6 years with Xolair; a 3-year withdrawal follow-up. Allergy. 2010;65:56–60.
119. Baena-Cagnani CE, Teijeiro A, Canonica GW. Four-year follow-up in children with moderate/severe uncontrolled asthma after withdrawal of a 1-year omalizumab treatment. Curr Opin Allergy Clin Immunol. 2015;15:267–71.
120. Kuprys-Lipinska I, Kuna P. Loss of asthma control after cessation of omalizumab treatment: real life data. Postepy Dermatol Alergol. 2014;31:1–5.
121. Solèr M. Omalizumab for severe allergic asthma: 7 years and open questions. Respiration. 2014;88:158–61.
122. Holgate ST, Djukanovich R, Casale T, et al. Anti-immunoglobulin E treatment with omalizumab in allergic diseases: an update on anti-inflammatory activity and clinical efficacy. Clin Exp Allergy. 2005;35:408–16.
123. Cox L, Platts-Mills TAE, Finegold I, et al. American Academy of Allergy, Asthma and Immunology/American College of Allergy, Asthma and Immunology Joint Task Force report on omalizumab-associated anaphylaxis. J Allergy Clin Immunol. 2007;120:1373–7.
124. Busse W, Buhl R, Fernandez Vidaurre C, et al. Omalizumab and the risk of malignancy: results from a pooled analysis. J Allergy Clin Immunol. 2012;129:983–9.
125. Long A, Rahmaoui A, Rothman KJ, et al. Incidence of malignancy in patients with moderate-to-severe asthma treated with or without omalizumab. J Allergy Clin Immunol. 2014;134:560–7.
126. Winchester DE, Jacob A, Murphy T. Omalizumab for asthma. N Engl J Med. 2006;355:1281–2.
127. Puéchal X, Rivereau P, Vinchon F. Churg-Strauss syndrome associated with omalizumab. Eur J Intern Med. 2008;19:364–6.
128. Bargagli E, Madioni C, Olivieri C, et al. Churg-Strauss vasculitis in a patient treated with omalizumab. J Asthma. 2008;45:115–6.
129. Vaglio A, Moosig F, Zwerina J. Churg-Strauss syndrome: update on pathophysiology and treatment. Curr Opin Rheumatol. 2012;24:24–30.
130. Cruz AA, Lima F, Sarinho E, et al. Safety of anti-immunoglobulin E therapy with omalizumab in allergic patients at risk of geohelminth infections. Clin Exp Allergy. 2007;37:197–207.
131. Corren J, Casale TB, Lanier B, et al. Safety and tolerability of omalizumab. Clin Exp Allergy. 2009;39:788–97.
132. Namazy J, Cabana MD, Scheuerle AE, et al. The Xolair Pregnancy Registry (EXPECT): the safety of omalizumab use during pregnancy. J Allergy Clin Immunol. 2015;135:407–12.
133. Tan RA, Corren J. Safety of omalizumab in asthma. Expert Opin Drug Saf. 2011;10:463–71.
134. Pelaia G, Renda T, Romeo P, et al. Omalizumab in the treatment of severe asthma: efficacy and current problems. Ther Adv Respir Dis. 2008;2:409–21.
135. Brown R, Turk F, Dale P, et al. Cost-effectiveness of omalizumab in patients with severe persistent allergic asthma. Allergy. 2007;62:149–53.
136. Oba Y, Salzman GA. Cost-effectiveness analysis of omalizumab in adults and adolescents with moderate-to-severe allergic asthma. J Allergy Clin Immunol. 2004;114:265–9.
137. Dewilde S, Turk F, Tambour M, et al. The economic value of anti-IgE in severe persistent, IgE-mediated (allergic) asthma patients: adaptation of INNOVATE to Sweden. Curr Med Res Opin. 2006;22:1765–76.
138. van Nooten F, Stern S, Braunstahl GJ, et al. Cost-effectiveness of omalizumab for uncontrolled allergic asthma in the Netherlands. J Med Econ. 2012;16:342–8.
139. Dal Negro RW, Pradelli L, Tognella S, et al. Cost utility of add-on omalizumab in difficult-to-treat allergic asthma in Italy. Eur Ann Allergy Clin Immunol. 2011;43:45–53.

140. Dal Negro RW, Tognella S, Pradelli L. A 36-month study on the cost/utility of add-on omalizumab in persistent difficult-to-treat atopic asthma in Italy. J Asthma. 2012;49:843–8.
141. Sullivan SD, Turk F. An evaluation of the cost-effectiveness of omalizumab for the treatment of severe allergic asthma. Allergy. 2008;63:670–84.
142. Arm JP, Bottoli I, Skerjanek A, et al. Pharmacokinetics, pharmacodynamics and safety of QGE031 (ligelizumab), a novel high-affinity anti-IgE antibody, in atopic subjects. Clin Exp Allergy. 2014;44:1371–85.
143. Menzella F, Lusuardi M, Galeone C, Zucchi L. Tailored therapy for severe asthma. Multidiscip Respir Med. 2015;10:1.
144. Nyborg AC, Zacco A, Ettinger R, et al. Development of an antibody that neutralizes soluble IgE and eliminates IgE expressing B-cells. Cell Mol Immunol. 2016;13:391–400.

IL-5-Targeted Antibodies

5

Because of the central role played by interleukin-5 (IL-5) in maturation, activation, proliferation and survival of eosinophils, this cytokine is a key target for treatment of eosinophilic asthma [1–4]. In this regard it is noteworthy that, among the pleiotropic effects of corticosteroids, inhibition of IL-5 synthesis is one of the most important mechanisms underlying the very effective antiasthma action of these drugs [5]. Corticosteroids are indeed powerful inducers of eosinophil apoptosis [6, 7]; nevertheless, despite a regular or almost continuous use of inhaled and even systemic corticosteroids, some subgroups of asthmatic subjects display persistent bronchial and/or blood eosinophilia, associated with an inadequate control of asthma [8]. Therefore, these patients can potentially benefit from additional therapies based on the use of biologic drugs targeting IL-5.

Role of IL-5 in Eosinophilic Asthma

IL-5 plays a pivotal pathogenic role in eosinophilic asthma. In asthmatic airways, the main cellular sources of IL-5 include Th2 lymphocytes, CD4+ invariant NK T cells, group 2 innate lymphoid cells (ILC2s), mast cells and eosinophils themselves [9–13]. Production of Th2 cytokines, also including IL-5, is markedly enhanced by IL-25 [14]. In patients with allergic asthma, the bone marrow is able to respond to allergen challenge with an enhanced capacity of producing eosinophils, and this effect is associated with higher concentrations of IL-5 mRNA in subjects experiencing dual early and late asthmatic responses, when compared to patients showing only early bronchoconstrictive reactions [15]. Besides its action exerted in the bone marrow, IL-5 seems to be capable of inducing eosinophil differentiation also inside the airways; indeed, increased levels of IL-5, eosinophil progenitors and mature eosinophils have been detected in the induced sputum of dual-responder asthmatics [16]. IL-5 synergizes with powerful eosinophil-chemotactic chemokines, namely, eotaxins 1, 2 and 3, in eliciting airway eosinophilia and bronchial hyperresponsiveness [3]. Furthermore, significantly increased sputum levels of IL-5 and eotaxins have been found in patients undergoing acute asthma exacerbations, when compared with both healthy controls and subjects with mild persistent disease [17]. IL-5 and eotaxins cooperate in favouring eosinophil accumulation into the airways, especially during asthma exacerbations, and this effect is at least in part dependent on IL-5-induced inhibition of eosinophil apoptosis [18, 19]. Sputum levels of IL-5

© Springer International Publishing Switzerland 2017   51
G. Pelaia et al., *Asthma: Targeted Biological Therapies*,
DOI 10.1007/978-3-319-46007-9_5

were indeed found to be inversely correlated with the numbers of apoptotic eosinophils in both stable and exacerbated asthmatic patients. Also in nonallergic, late-onset eosinophilic asthma, IL-5 exerts a key pathogenic role [20]. In this particular asthmatic phenotype, large amounts of IL-5 are produced by ILC2s [21] in the absence of active allergic pathways triggered by Th2 lymphocytes.

On eosinophils, the cellular effects of IL-5 are mediated by its binding to a membrane receptor including a ligand-specific α subunit (IL-5Rα) and a nonspecific signalling βc subunit (Fig. 5.1), which also interacts via a shared extracellular domain with two other haematopoietic cytokines such as interleukin-3 (IL-3) and granulocyte-macrophage colony-stimulating factor (GM-CSF) [23, 24]. High-affinity binding of IL-5 to IL-5Rα is followed by ligation of this IL-5-/IL-5Rα-activated complex to the βc subunit, which probably triggers signal transduction via dimerization of its cytoplasmic domain [25, 26]. The signalling pathways activated by the interaction of IL-5 with its receptor involve several transducing enzymes (Fig. 5.1), mainly including intracellular kinases such as Janus kinases (JAK), mitogen-activated protein kinases, Lyn tyrosine kinase, Raf-1 kinase and phosphoinositide 3-kinase [3].

Independently of IL-5, JAK2 and JAK1 are constitutively associated with IL-5Rα and the βc chain, respectively [27]. Upon IL-5 binding, the receptor structural construct undergoes a dynamic conformational change, leading to the association of JAK1 with IL-5Rα [27]. Therefore, IL-5 activates both JAK1 and JAK2, thus triggering the assembly of a functional IL-5Rα-βc complex. As a result of this

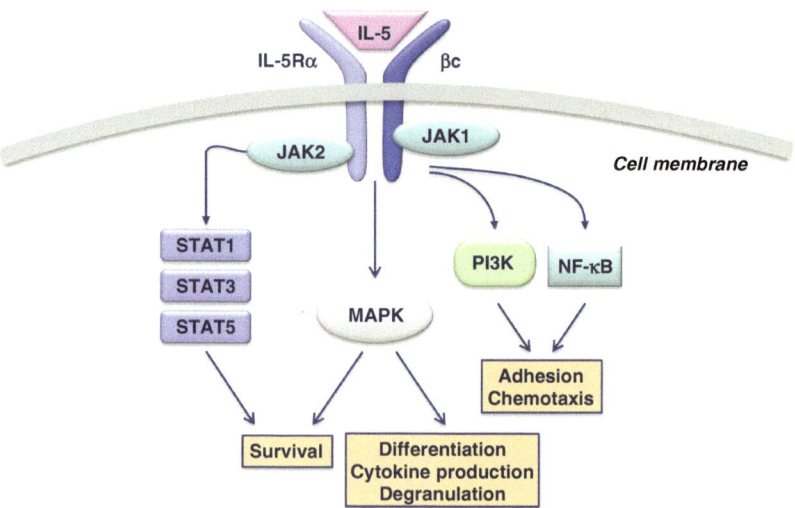

Fig. 5.1 Molecular mechanisms and signalling pathways activated by IL-5 in eosinophils. Binding of IL-5 to the α subunit of its receptor (IL-5Rα) induces the assembly of a dimeric receptor complex consisting of both α and βc subunits. The subsequent activation of several signalling pathways, including JAK/STAT, MAPK, PI3K and NF-kB, is responsible for transcription of genes involved in eosinophil differentiation, degranulation, survival, proliferation, chemotaxis and adhesion. See text for further details (Reprinted from Ref. [22])

IL-5-dependent stimulatory process, JAK2 induces the activation of signal trans-ducers and activators of transcription (STAT) 1, 3 and 5, which enhance the expression of pim-1, cyclin D3 and other IL-5-inducible genes involved in cell cycle progression and eosinophil proliferation [28, 29]. JAK2 is also implicated, via a cooperative action with Lyn and Raf-1 kinases, in IL-5-mediated inhibition of eosinophil apoptosis, thereby contributing to cell survival [30]. Moreover, Raf-1 plays a key role in eosinophil activation and degranulation [30].

Within the context of the intricate IL-5-stimulated signalling network activated by the βc receptor subunit, a central role is played by both ERK and p38 subgroups of mitogen-activated protein kinases (MAPK). In particular, Ras/Raf-1/MEK-mediated activation of ERK is crucially responsible for induction of *c-fos* gene expression and eosinophil differentiation, proliferation and survival, as well as for the release of leukotriene C_4 [31–34]. Furthermore, p38 MAPK mainly induces, also acting through activation of the transcription factor NF-kB, cytokine production by eosinophils, and eosinophil adhesion and chemotaxis occurring during allergic inflammation [34–36]. IL-5-induced adhesion of eosinophils to intercellular adhesion molecule-1 (ICAM-1) is also promoted by phosphoinositide 3-kinase (PI3K), and this effect is mediated by downstream stimulation of protein kinase C (PKC) and phosphorylation-dependent activation of ERK1/2 [37].

Given the pivotal role played by IL-5 in eosinophil functions and asthma pathobiology, this cytokine and its receptor are suitable targets of biological therapies undergoing evaluation for treatment of eosinophilic asthma [38]. In this regard, several preclinical studies have been carried out in experimental animal models of asthma. Indeed, the anti-IL-5 antibody TRFK-5 suppressed airway eosinophilia in allergen-sensitized mice [39]. Moreover, in nonhuman primate models of asthma, TRFK-5 inhibited the influx of eosinophils into bronchi and the associated airway hyperresponsiveness [40]. Later, other monoclonal antibodies directed against IL-5 (mepolizumab and reslizumab) or IL-5Rα (benralizumab) have been developed and evaluated in clinical trials (Fig. 5.2) [41–43].

Mepolizumab

Mepolizumab (SB-240563) is a humanized IgG1/k monoclonal antibody which selectively binds with high affinity to IL-5 (Fig. 5.2), thus preventing its interaction with IL-5Rα [44–46]. In particular, mepolizumab was generated by grafting antihuman IL-5 antigen recognition sites from murine origin onto a human IgG1 heavy chain [47]. Some early clinical trials, carried out in heterogeneous populations of patients with mild or moderate chronic persistent asthma, showed that mepolizumab significantly decreased eosinophil numbers in both blood and induced sputum [48–50]. However, these effects were not associated with relevant changes in asthma symptoms, lung function, bronchial hyperresponsiveness and activation status of T lymphocytes. In particular, administered at a single intravenous dose of 10 mg/kg, mepolizumab did not improve the late asthmatic reaction to allergen challenge and the bronchial response to histamine in subjects with mild asthma [48]. Furthermore,

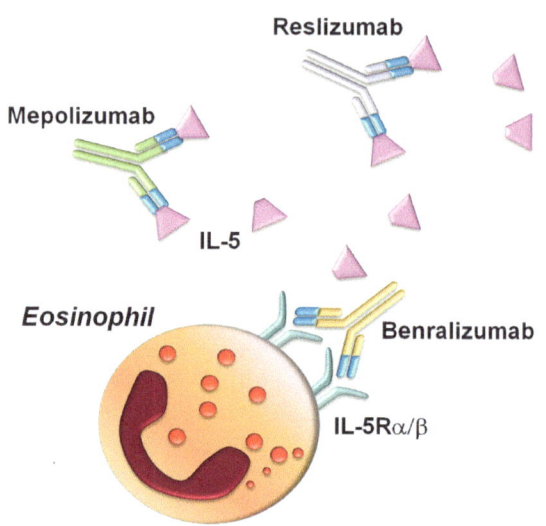

in patients with moderate persistent asthma receiving a monthly intravenous dose of 250 or 750 mg for 3 months, mepolizumab did not lower exacerbation rates, did not increase either forced expiratory volume in 1 s (FEV_1) or peak expiratory flow (PEF) and did not improve the overall quality of life (QoL) [49].

Subsequently, mepolizumab was evaluated by Haldar et al. and Nair et al. in small groups of subjects with carefully selected phenotypes of chronic severe asthma, characterized by recurrent exacerbations and bronchial eosinophilia refractory to both inhaled and systemic corticosteroids [51, 52]. Taken together, the results of these two small targeted trials showed that mepolizumab effectively reduced asthma exacerbations and eosinophil levels in both blood and induced sputum. In addition to these effects, given at a monthly intravenous dosage of 750 mg for 4 months, mepolizumab also significantly decreased prednisone consumption and slightly enhanced FEV_1 values [52]. Further important information was gained by the longer study conducted by Haldar and colleagues [51]. In this trial, mepolizumab was delivered for 1 year through 12 monthly intravenous infusions of 750 mg. Chest imaging performed by computed tomography (CT) scans obtained before and after treatment demonstrated that when compared with placebo, mepolizumab significantly reduced airway wall thickness and total wall area [51]. Therefore, these results suggest that mepolizumab can possibly affect bronchial remodelling, an airway structural feature which is especially relevant in severe asthma. Such findings thus confirmed previous observations reported by Flood-Page et al., who showed that mepolizumab was able to decrease the deposition of extracellular matrix proteins in the reticular basement membrane of bronchial mucosa and also to reduce the levels of transforming growth factor-β1 (TGF-β1) in bronchoalveolar lavage fluid (BALF) [53]. Hence, the potential anti-remodelling action of mepolizumab is very likely due to its capability of depleting eosinophils, which are prominent cellular sources of TGF-β1, one of the most important growth factors contributing to airway structural changes in asthma [54].

The results obtained by Haldar and Nair have been further corroborated by the large, multicentre, phase 2b/3 Dose Ranging Efficacy And safety with Mepolizumab in severe asthma (DREAM) study, carried out by Pavord et al. in more than 600 patients with severe, exacerbation-prone and eosinophilic asthma, who were randomly assigned to four groups receiving at 4-week intervals 13 intravenous infusions of placebo or one of three doses of mepolizumab (75 mg, 250 mg or 750 mg) [55]. At all dosages used, mepolizumab effectively lowered blood and sputum eosinophil counts, as well as the frequency of asthma exacerbations by 39–52%, regardless of IgE levels and atopic status [55]. However, no significant improvements in either asthma symptoms or lung function were detected. Interestingly, the enrolment criteria of this trial were based on the presence of a blood eosinophil count higher than 300 cells/microlitre. Indeed, this inclusion parameter is easily and routinely measurable, thereby being much better assessable than the rather complex-to-perform cellular analysis of induced sputum, often not feasible in a real-life setting because of obvious requirements for a greater extent of technical and interpretative expertise. The results of the DREAM trial are consistent with those of a recent meta-analysis, referring to seven randomized and placebo-controlled studies, which investigated the effects of intravenous mepolizumab, thus concluding that this anti-IL-5 antibody decreased the risk of exacerbations and improved QoL in patients with eosinophilic asthma but did not significantly affect symptoms and lung function [56].

In 2014, the results of two other trials were published about the efficacy of mepolizumab in patients with severe eosinophilic asthma, experiencing more than two exacerbations in the previous year despite the use of high doses of inhaled corticosteroids, associated with additional antiasthma drugs. In particular, the double-blind phase 3 SteroId ReductIon with mepolizUmab Study (SIRIUS) was carried out by Bel et al. in 135 patients with severe eosinophilic asthma requiring a daily oral corticosteroid therapy as maintenance treatment for at least 6 months, who were randomly assigned to receive either placebo or a low subcutaneous dose (100 mg) of mepolizumab every 4 weeks for 20 weeks [57]. When compared with placebo, mepolizumab provided an oral glucocorticoid-sparing effect consisting of a 50% reduction in prednisone consumption. Moreover, mepolizumab also lowered asthma exacerbations and improved QoL and symptom control. The larger MEpolizumab as adjunctive therapy iNpatients with Severe Asthma (MENSA) study was conducted by Ortega et al., who recruited 576 subjects with severe eosinophilic asthma on treatment with high doses of inhaled corticosteroids, aged between 12 and 82 years, and experiencing at least two exacerbations during the previous year, which required a systemic glucocorticoid therapy [58]. Furthermore, the enrolled patients were characterized by FEV_1 values lower than 80 and 90% predicted for adults and adolescents under the age of 18 years, respectively. Other study requirements included FEV_1 reversibility of more than 12%, FEV_1 variability $\geq 20\%$ between two clinic visits in the past 12 months and a positive response to a bronchial challenge with either methacholine or mannitol during the previous year. In comparison with placebo, administration of mepolizumab every 4 weeks for 32 weeks, at dosages of 75 mg intravenously or 100 mg subcutaneously, induced significant decreases in asthma exacerbation rates of either 47% or 53%, respectively. Moreover, both drug doses elicited significant improvements in QoL. Similar to the SIRIUS study, also the MENSA trial documented a modest FEV_1 increase [57, 58]. Post hoc analyses of both SIRIUS and MENSA studies have recently shown, in patients with severe eosinophilic asthma, that mepolizumab treatment was effective in decreasing disease exacerbations and improving asthma control and quality of life, regardless of previous use of omalizumab [59].

All these trials outlined a very good profile of safety and tolerability for mepolizumab, which resulted to be similar to placebo with regard to side effects and adverse events [46, 60]. The most common adverse events occurring during SIRIUS and MENSA studies were headache and nasopharyngitis [57, 58]. In addition, during the MENSA trial, a slightly higher percentage of injection-site reactions was observed using mepolizumab subcutaneously (9%), with respect to intravenous administration (3%) [58]. The development of neutralizing anti-mepolizumab antibodies is a very rare event, which has been only sporadically reported [61]. The long-term safety of mepolizumab was also confirmed by an open-label study performed in 78 patients with hypereosinophilic syndromes, who experienced a good drug tolerance throughout a mean treatment period of 251 weeks [62].

On the basis of the convincing evidence inferred from all these studies, in November 2015 mepolizumab became the first anti-cytokine biologic drug to be approved by the US Food and Drug Administration (FDA) as an add-on maintenance treatment for severe asthmatic patients, aged 12 years and older, with a documented eosinophilic phenotype. Furthermore, mepolizumab has been recently included within the step 5 of Global Initiative for Asthma (GINA) guidelines, as add-on therapy for severe eosinophilic asthma, uncontrolled by standard treatments [63].

Reslizumab

Reslizumab is an IgG4/k monoclonal antibody, also known as SCH-55700, which was humanized from the rat monoclonal IgG2a antibody JES1-39D10 via a synthetic process based on recombinant technology using complementarity-determining region grafting, aimed to incorporate rat antigen recognition sites for human IL-5 onto a human IgG4 structure [22, 64–66]. Reslizumab has a molecular weight of 146 kDa and binds with high affinity to an epitope region corresponding to amino acids 89–92 of human IL-5, thus preventing this cytokine from binding to IL-5Rα (Fig. 5.2) [67–69].

The first clinical study aimed to assess the efficacy of reslizumab in asthma treatment was carried out by Kips et al. in a small group of asthmatic subjects [70]. This phase 2, double-blind, randomized and dose-ranging pilot trial evaluated the biological, clinical and functional effects, as well as the safety and pharmacokinetic profiles, of reslizumab. Enrolled patients were recruited on the basis of their severe persistent asthma, treated with oral glucocorticoids or high doses of inhaled corticosteroids, regardless of the underlying inflammatory phenotypes. Reslizumab was compared with placebo ($n=8$) and administered as a single intravenous infusion at four rising doses of 0.03 mg/kg ($n=2$), 0.1 mg/kg ($n=4$), 0.3 mg/kg ($n=6$) or 1.0 mg/kg ($n=12$), respectively. When compared with placebo, at doses ≥ 0.3 mg/kg, reslizumab significantly reduced eosinophil counts in peripheral blood with respect to baseline values, thus inducing mean decreases in circulating eosinophils ranging from 52.5 % at 48 h to 18.9 % at day 30. Moreover, reslizumab lowered sputum eosinophil numbers in three of four patients with documented bronchial eosinophilia. However, no significant changes were detected in both symptom control and physician evaluation of overall clinical status. With regard to lung function, in comparison with placebo, reslizumab elicited a transiently significant increase in FEV_1, recorded 24 h after administration of the 0.3 mg/kg dosage. Although a trend towards FEV_1 improvement also persisted at subsequent time points, no dose of reslizumab was able to induce further significant FEV_1 changes. On day 30, FEV_1 increases with respect to baseline values were 11.2 % in the 0.3 mg/kg group, 8.6 % in the 1.0 mg/kg arm and 4.0 % in patients assigned to placebo treatment. Furthermore, no meaningful variations were observed in terms of either FEV_1/forced vital capacity (FEV_1/FVC) ratio or peak expiratory flow (PEF). With regard to safety, all single doses of reslizumab were well tolerated, and no significant alterations of vital signs or laboratory parameters were found. The most common adverse events included headache and fatigue, which were reported with the same frequency also in the placebo group. Similarly, no significant differences were detected with regard to asthma worsening, which occurred in 3 of 12 patients treated with 1.0 mg/kg of reslizumab and in 1 of 8 subjects of the placebo arm. In one patient treated with the dosage of 1.0 mg/kg, non-neutralizing serum antibodies to reslizumab were found. The plasma levels of reslizumab were dose proportional. At 6.9 h after administration of the 1.0 mg/kg dose, the pharmacokinetic profile of reslizumab was characterized by a mean maximal concentration of 30.3 micrograms/ml. After the same drug dosage, mean concentrations of 0.87 and 0.43 micrograms/ml were detected on days 90 and 120, respectively. The elimination half-life ranged between 24.5 and 30.1 days.

Later, in a phase 2 multicentre, double-blind study performed in Northern America (the USA and Canada) and specifically targeted to eosinophilic asthma, Castro et al. evaluated the effects of reslizumab in 106 patients with inadequately controlled disease despite the use of high doses of inhaled corticosteroids [71]. Patient enrolment was made on the basis of an eosinophil percentage of at least 3 % in induced sputum. In particular, 53 subjects were randomly assigned to treatment with placebo, and the other 53 patients were treated with four intravenous infusions of 3.0 mg/kg of reslizumab, administered every 4 weeks for 12 weeks, respectively. With respect to baseline counts, at the end of treatment, reslizumab induced a significant, median 95.4 % reduction of sputum eosinophils. In clinical terms, this effect was associated with a positive trend towards better asthma control, which however did not reach the threshold of statistical significance; greater improvements in asthma control were achieved by a subgroup of patients characterized by the highest levels of blood and sputum eosinophils, associated with nasal polyposis. In comparison with placebo, a positive but not significant difference in favour of the reslizumab arm was also observed in the rate of asthma exacerbations. With regard to lung function, when compared to placebo, reslizumab elicited significant improvements in both FEV_1 (mean FEV_1 increase, 180 ml) and FVC. This trial confirmed the good tolerability profile of reslizumab. Indeed, in reslizumab and placebo arms, the proportions of patients who experienced adverse events were very similar. The most frequently reported adverse event was nasopharyngitis.

More recently, two large, multicentre, double-blind, randomized and placebo-controlled, phase 3 trials have been carried out by Castro et al. with the primary end point of evaluating the effects of reslizumab on asthma exacerbations in patients with poorly controlled disease and blood eosinophilia [72]. Inclusion criteria were based on the occurrence of one or more exacerbations treated with systemic corticosteroids during the previous year, associated with blood eosinophil counts ≥ 400 cells/microlitre and with an inadequate asthma control despite the use of medium-to-high doses of inhaled corticosteroids, eventually utilized with the addition of other drugs including long-acting β_2 adrenergic agonists, leukotriene modifiers, cromolyn sodium and even oral glucocorticoids. Recruited patients continued their usual asthma therapies at constant doses throughout both studies. Among 2597 patients screened, 953 were enrolled and randomly assigned to receive intravenous infusions of either placebo or reslizumab, administered at a dosage of 3.0 mg/kg every 4 weeks for 52 weeks. When compared with placebo, reslizumab significantly lowered the annual rate of clinical asthma exacerbations by 50–59 %. Reslizumab also prolonged the time to first exacerbation. Moreover, in both trials reslizumab significantly decreased blood eosinophil numbers, improved asthma symptom control and increased FEV_1 values. These two parallel trials confirmed the good safety profile of reslizumab, which resulted to be similar to that of placebo [72]. In both studies, the most commonly reported adverse events, occurring in more than 5 % of patients receiving reslizumab, were worsening of asthma symptoms, nasopharyngitis, upper respiratory tract infections, sinusitis, influenza and headache. Overall, when compared with subjects treated with placebo, serious adverse events were less frequent in patients receiving reslizumab. Local reactions at injection sites resulted to be uncommon and not different between placebo and reslizumab arms. In study 2, two patients receiving reslizumab experienced anaphylactic reactions, which responded well to standard treatment, but led to withdrawal from the trial; antidrug antibodies (ADA) were not detected in both subjects. Transient, low-titre anti-reslizumab antibodies were found in eight patients (3 %) in study 1 and in seven patients (2 %) in study 2, respectively. However, in these subjects the overall safety pattern of reslizumab did not result to be different from that globally recorded in both study populations.

The positive effects on lung function, mainly referring to enlargement of proximal airways, can be integrated by further improvements also occurring at the level of peripheral airways as shown by another phase 3 study conducted by Bjermer et al. [73]. In particular, the results of this trial, aimed to evaluate the effects of two different dosages (0.3 and 3.0 mg/kg) of intravenous reslizumab, refer to 311 patients with persistent asthma, reversible airflow limitation and high levels of blood eosinophils (≥ 400 cells/microlitre), not adequately controlled by inhaled corticosteroids. At the end of the first part of this investigation, 271 patients chosen among those receiving either drug ($n = 179$) or placebo ($n = 92$) were enrolled into an open-label extension study and received the 3.0 mg/kg dose of reslizumab. When compared to placebo after 16 weeks of treatment, both dosages of reslizumab induced significant increases in mean FEV_1 values (115 and 160 mL with 0.3 and 3 mg/kg, respectively). Furthermore, only when administered at the 3.0 mg/kg dose, reslizumab also elicited significant increases in mean values of both FVC (130 ml) and forced expiratory flow at 25–75 % of FVC ($FEF_{25-75\%}$) (233 ml/s). At both dosages (0.3 and 3.0 mg/kg), reslizumab improved symptom control evaluated through Asthma Control Questionnaire (ACQ) score, as well as decreased the use of inhaled rescue medications. Additionally, although both reslizumab doses significantly lowered blood eosinophil counts, a greater effect was observed when the 3 mg/kg dose was used. Treatment with reslizumab at both dosages was well tolerated, and only mild-to-moderate and self-limiting adverse events related to the study drug, including headache, nasopharyngitis, upper respiratory tract infections and sinusitis, were recorded. Low anti-drug antibodies (ADA) titres were detected in 12 and 11 % of patients treated with reslizumab 0.3 mg/kg and 3 mg/kg, respectively. However, the majority of these patients resulted to be ADA positive only once during the 16-week treatment period. Moreover, the safety profile of ADA-positive patients was similar to that observed in the global study population, and ADA positivity did not have any impact on blood eosinophil suppression operated by reslizumab, thus suggesting that ADAs were not neutralizing [73].

The above-mentioned data were indirectly confirmed by a further phase 3 study performed by Corren et al., who completed their analysis in 492 patients with poorly controlled asthma, not selected on the basis of their blood eosinophil counts, who over a period of 16 weeks received every 4 weeks placebo ($n = 97$) or 3.0 mg/kg of intravenous reslizumab ($n = 395$) [74]. The authors did not report significant changes in FEV_1 in the overall study population and in the subgroup of patients with less than 400 blood eosinophils/microlitre. However, in the subgroup of patients with more than 400 blood eosinophils/microlitre, with respect to placebo, reslizumab produced a significant mean FEV_1 increase (270 mL). Reslizumab was well tolerated, and patients receiving this drug experienced fewer overall adverse events when compared with subjects assigned to the placebo arm (55 % versus 73 %). Low and transient ADA titres were detected in 5 % of patients treated with reslizumab, but ADA positivity did not affect either safety profile or eosinophil depletion pattern, thereby indicating a lack of neutralizing activity [74].

The use of reslizumab for the maintenance treatment of patients suffering from severe uncontrolled asthma has been recently approved by the FDA.

Benralizumab

Benralizumab (MEDI-563) is a humanized afucosylated IgG1k monoclonal antibody of murine origin, directed against the α subunit of IL-5R (Fig. 5.2) expressed by both eosinophils and basophils [75]. In particular, benralizumab selectively recognizes an extracellular IL-5Rα epitope which is located very closely to the IL-5 binding site, thereby effectively inhibiting IL-5-dependent cell proliferation. In addition to neutralizing the key survival signal for eosinophils provided by IL-5, benralizumab induces eosinophil apoptosis also through antibody-dependent cell-mediated cytotoxicity (ADCC) [76]. Indeed, elimination of the fucose sugar residue in the CH2 region of the oligosaccharide core of human IgG1 elicited a five- to 50-fold increase in the antibody affinity for the Fcγ receptor (human FcγRIIIa) present on the surface of natural killer (NK) cells, macrophages and neutrophils [77, 78]. Such an enhanced binding affinity of benralizumab for these cells resulted in a ≥1000-fold amplification, with respect to the parental fucosylated antibody, of eosinophil and basophil death induced via ADCC and dependent on the interaction with activating FcγRIIIa receptors [79].

In a phase 1, dose-rising study performed by Busse et al., pharmacokinetics and pharmacodynamics of benralizumab were assessed by monitoring blood eosinophil levels over 12 weeks after administration to patients with mild asthma of single, intravenous drug dosages included within a range of 0.0003–3 mg/kg [80]. Benralizumab persistently and dose-dependently depleted peripheral blood eosinophils. In particular, benralizumab-induced eosinopenia lasted at least 8 or 12 weeks with doses of 0.03–0.1 and 0.3–3 mg/kg, respectively, whereas blood eosinophil counts were not lowered by dosages ranging from 0.0003–0.003 mg/Kg. At doses of 0.03–3 mg/kg, the mean maximum concentration (1–82 micrograms/ml) was approximately dose proportional. The mean volume of distribution (52–93 ml/kg) of benralizumab was larger than the plasma volume, thereby indicating a possible binding to IL-5Rα-expressing blood cells, as well as a moderate penetration into extravascular tissues. The mean elimination half-life was approximately 2–3 weeks, which is typical of human IgG antibodies.

A subsequent phase 1, multicentre, randomized, double-blind and placebo-controlled study was conducted by Laviolette et al. and completed by 26 asthmatic patients, recruited on the basis of a documented bronchial hyperresponsiveness or reversible airway obstruction [81]. A single intravenous dose of 1 mg/kg of benralizumab was administered to eight patients, who were compared with five placebo-treated subjects. Furthermore, three monthly subcutaneous doses of placebo or 200 mg or 100 mg of benralizumab were delivered to four, five and four patients, respectively. Bronchoscopies with airway mucosal/submucosal biopsies were performed at baseline, and 28 days after end of treatment, with the aim of examining tissue eosinophils. Moreover, blood samples were taken to measure peripheral eosinophil counts. In a subgroup of patients, eosinophils were also analysed in induced sputum and bone marrow biopsies. After treatments with either intravenous or subcutaneous benralizumab, circulating eosinophils were not detectable anymore. Depletion of eosinophils and eosinophil precursors resulted to be complete also in bone marrow. In comparison to placebo, benralizumab also reduced eosinophil numbers in induced sputum and airway mucosal/submucosal biopsies; however, these decreases did not reach the threshold of statistical significance for each independent dosing. Therefore, such results suggest that while in bone marrow benralizumab was able to completely suppress the production of eosinophils, thus effectively removing these cells from bloodstream, the drug was less effective on eosinophils which had already reached the airways. Hence, it can be speculated that tissue eosinophils are possibly at a more advanced maturation stage, which makes them less susceptible to pharmacological treatments, also including anti-IL-5 therapies [82].

A phase 2a trial has been recently performed on patients having $\geq 2\%$ sputum eosinophils or FeNO ≥ 50 ppb (parts per billion), who had experienced 2–6 asthma exacerbations in the previous year, despite the use of medium/high doses of inhaled corticosteroids and long-acting β_2-adrenergic agonists [83]. 106 subjects were randomly subdivided into four groups, assigned to receive subcutaneous injections of placebo ($n=27$) or benralizumab at dosages of 2 mg ($n=27$), 20 mg ($n=26$) and 100 mg ($n=26$), respectively. Placebo or drug administrations were made on weeks 0 (day 1), 4, 8, 16, 24, 32 and 40. In comparison with placebo, at week 52 benralizumab reduced the annual exacerbation rates by 33, 45 or 36% when used at doses of 2, 20 or 100 mg, respectively. Furthermore, FEV_1 increased throughout the study period at all dosages of benralizumab, reaching the highest changes at week 52 after the 100 mg dose, especially in subjects with a blood eosinophil count ≥ 300 cells/ microlitre (mean FEV_1 increase: 28.1%). This drug also induced a remarkable decrease in peripheral blood eosinophil numbers. The safety profiles of all benralizumab doses were acceptable and did not significantly differed from placebo [83].

Benralizumab was also tested in a phase 2b randomized, dose-ranging trial, carried out by Castro et al. in patients with uncontrolled asthma [84]. This study was completed by 324 eosinophilic and 282 non-eosinophilic uncontrolled asthmatic patients, respectively, who had experienced from two to six asthma exacerbations during the previous year, despite a regular treatment with medium-high doses of inhaled corticosteroids, associated with long-acting β_2-adrenergic agonists. Of 324 eosinophilic subjects, 80 were randomly assigned to treatment with placebo, whereas other 81, 81 and 82 patients received 2 mg, 20 mg and 100 mg of benralizumab, respectively. With regard to 282 non-eosinophilic subjects, 142 received placebo and 140 were given 100 mg of benralizumab. Study drugs were administered as two subcutaneous injections every 4 weeks for the first three doses (weeks 1, 4 and 8) and then every 8 weeks (weeks 16, 24, 32 and 40). In comparison to placebo, at week 52 the annual rates of asthma exacerbations resulted to be lower in eosinophilic patients receiving 100 mg, but not 20 mg or 2 mg of benralizumab. This drug was more effective in decreasing exacerbations when blood eosinophil counts were ≥ 300 cells/microlitre. In these same patients, asthma exacerbations were reduced by benralizumab at both dosages of 100 and 20 mg. In non-eosinophilic individuals, 100 mg of benralizumab did not change the annual rate of asthma exacerbations. In eosinophilic asthmatics, all benralizumab doses decreased blood eosinophil numbers, improved asthma control and increased FEV_1 values. Mild-to-moderate adverse events were slightly more frequent in benralizumab groups than in placebo arms, with nasopharyngitis and local reactions at injection sites being the most commonly reported manifestations.

A further phase 2 study has been conducted by Nowak et al. who evaluated the effects, on recurrence of asthma exacerbations and/or on hospitalization for acute asthma, of a single intravenous infusion of benralizumab, added to current standard treatments prescribed on discharge from the emergency department [85]. This trial was completed by three subject groups, each consisting of 36 patients who randomly received placebo (first group) or benralizumab at a dosage of 0.3 mg/kg (second group) or 1.0 mg/kg (third group), respectively. Enrolled patients were chosen because, in addition to the occurrence of at least one previous exacerbation requiring an urgent care visit during the past 12 months, they presented to an emergency department for acute asthma and experienced only a partial response to treatment. In comparison to placebo, the effects induced by benralizumab 12 weeks after drug administration resulted in significant 49 and 60% reductions of asthma exacerbation rates and exacerbations leading to hospitalization, respectively. At the same time point, such findings were paralleled by remarkable decreases in blood eosinophil counts, as well as in serum levels of eosinophilic cationic protein and eosinophil-derived neurotoxin, which are important markers of cell activation. All these effects were observed after injection of both 0.3 and 1.0 mg/kg doses of benralizumab. This drug displayed a good safety profile. Indeed, only mild-to-moderate and self-limiting adverse events were observed, including headache, dizziness, cough, fever, bronchitis, anxiety, muscle spasms and hyperhidrosis. At week 12, anti-benralizumab antibodies were detected in six patients, who however did not experience any clinical consequence.

Concluding Remarks

The well-established awareness of the role of IL-5 as a key player in the pathobiology of eosinophilic asthma has promoted the development of effective therapeutic strategies aimed to neutralize this cytokine or to block its receptor (Fig. 5.2) [86]. Indeed, as a result of several randomized controlled trials, most of them already completed and some currently ongoing, mepolizumab, reslizumab and benralizumab will probably be introduced in clinical practice in a not too far away future. Of course, a focused selection of eligible asthmatic patients for anti-IL-5 biotherapies requires a careful phenotypic stratification, based on reliable clinical, functional and biologic features. In particular, subjects who can take the best advantages from the use of biologic drugs targeting IL-5 or its receptor are likely those suffering from uncontrolled eosinophilic, allergic or nonallergic asthma, also experiencing recurrent disease exacerbations despite the use of inhaled corticosteroids at relatively high doses. Of course, the most important biomarkers of eosinophilic airway inflammation are sputum eosinophils. However, because of the practical unfeasibility of induced sputum in many clinical settings of real-life routine medical activity, peripheral blood eosinophils represent a very useful and easily measurable parameter in order to characterize these patients. Indeed, the levels of circulating eosinophils approximately reflect, even better than fractioned exhaled nitric oxide, the state of ongoing bronchial inflammation [87–89]. Therefore, it seems very reasonable that anti-IL-5 add-on treatments will soon contribute to satisfy the unmet needs of patients with moderate-to-severe eosinophilic asthma, not adequately controlled by current standard therapies.

References

1. Weltman JK, Karim AS. IL-5: biology and potential therapeutic applications. Expert Opin Investig Drugs. 2000;9:491–6.
2. Stirling RG, van Rensen EI, Barnes PJ, Chung KF. Interleukin-5 induces CD34+ eosinophil progenitor mobilization and eosinophil CCR3 expression in asthma. Am J Respir Crit Care Med. 2001;164:1403–9.
3. Molfino NA, Gossage D, Kolbeck R, et al. Molecular and clinical rationale for therapeutic targeting of interleukin-5 and its receptor. Clin Exp Allergy. 2012;42:712–37.
4. Fulkerson PC, Rothenberg ME. Targeting eosinophils in allergy, inflammation and beyond. Nat Rev Drug Discov. 2013;12:117–29.
5. Barnes PJ, Adcock IM. How do corticosteroids work in asthma? Ann Intern Med. 2003;139:359–70.
6. Zhang X, Moilanen E, Kankaanranta H. Enhancement of human eosinophil apoptosis by fluticasone propionate, budesonide, and beclomethasone. Eur J Pharmacol. 2000;406:325–32.
7. Zhang X, Moilanen E, Adcock IM, et al. Divergent effect of mometasone on human eosinophil and neutrophil apoptosis. Life Sci. 2002;71:1523–34.
8. Barnes PJ. Corticosteroid resistance in patients with asthma and chronic obstructive pulmonary disease. J Allergy Clin Immunol. 2013;131:636–45.
9. Woodruff PG, Modrek B, Choy DF, et al. T-helper type 2-driven inflammation defines major sub-phenotypes of asthma. Am J Respir Crit Care Med. 2009;180:388–95.
10. Sakuishi K, Oki S, Araki M, et al. Invariant NKT cells biased for IL-5 production act as crucial regulators of inflammation. J Immunol. 2007;179:3452–62.
11. Yu S, Kim HY, Chang YJ, et al. Innate lymphoid cells and asthma. J Allergy Clin Immunol. 2014;133:943–50.
12. Shakoory B, Fitzgerald SM, Lee SA, et al. The role of human mast cell-derived cytokines in eosinophil biology. J Interferon Cytokine Res. 2004;24:271–81.
13. Hogan SP, Rosenberg HF, Moqbel R, et al. Eosinophils: biological properties and role in health and disease. Clin Exp Allergy. 2009;38:709–50.
14. Wang YH, Liu YJ. Thymic stromal lymphopoietin, OX40-ligand, and interleukin-25 in allergic responses. Clin Exp Allergy. 2009;39:798–806.
15. Wood LJ, Sehmi R, Dorman S, et al. Allergen-induced increases in bone marrow T lymphocytes and interleukin-5 expression in subjects with asthma. Am J Respir Crit Care Med. 2002;166:883–9.
16. Dorman SC, Efthimiadis A, Babirad I, et al. Sputum CD34+ IL-5Rα+cells increase after allergen: evidence for in situ eosinophilopoiesis. Am J Respir Crit Care Med. 2004;169:573–7.
17. Park SW, Kim DJ, Chang HS, et al. Association of interleukin-5 and eotaxin with acute exacerbation of asthma. Int Arch Allergy Immunol. 2003;131:283–90.
18. Xu J, Jiang F, Nayeri F, Zetterstrom O. Apoptotic eosinophils in sputum from asthmatic patients correlate negatively with levels of IL-5 and eotaxin. Respir Med. 2007;101:1447–54.
19. Ilmarinen P, Moilanen E, Kankaanranta H. Regulation of spontaneous eosinophil apoptosis – a neglected area of importance. J Cell Death. 2014;7:1–9.
20. Brusselle GG, Maes T, Bracke KR. Eosinophilic airway inflammation in nonallergic asthma. Nat Med. 2013;19:977–9.
21. Walker JA, Barlow JL, McKenzie AM. Innate lymphoid cells: how did we miss them? Nat Rev Immunol. 2013;13:75–87.
22. Pelaia G, Vatrella A, Busceti MT, et al. Role of biologics in severe eosinophilic asthma – focus on reslizumab. Ther Clin Risk Manag 2016;12:1075–1082.
23. Rossjohn J, McKinstry WJ, Woodcock JM, et al. Structure of the activation domain of the GM-CSF/IL-3/IL-5 receptor common β-chain bound to an antagonist. Blood. 2000;95:2491–8.
24. Murphy JM, Young IG. IL-3, IL-5, and GM-CSF signaling: crystal structure of the human β-common receptor. Vitam Horm. 2006;74:1–30.

25. Johanson K, Appelbaum E, Doyle M, et al. Binding interactions of human interleukin 5 with its receptor α subunit. Large scale production, structural, and functional studies of Drosophila-expressed recombinant proteins. J Biol Chem. 1995;270:9459–71.
26. Ishino T, Harrington AE, Gopi H, Chaiken I. Structure-based rationale for interleukin 5 receptor antagonism. Curr Pharm Des. 2008;14:1231–9.
27. Kouro T, Takatsu K. IL-5- and eosinophil-mediated inflammation: from discovery to therapy. Int Immunol. 2009;21:1303–9.
28. Pazdrak K, Stafford S, Alam R. The activation of the Jak-STAT 1 signalling pathway by IL-5 in eosinophils. J Immunol. 1995;155:397–402.
29. Stout BA, Bates ME, Liu LY, et al. IL-5 and granulocyte-macrophage colony-stimulating factor activate STAT3 and STAT5 and promote Pim-1 and cyclin D3 protein expression in human eosinophils. J Immunol. 2004;173:6409–17.
30. Pazdrak K, Olszewska-Pazdrak B, Stafford S, et al. Lyn, Jak2, and Raf-1 kinases are critical for the antiapoptotic effect of interleukin-5, whereas only Raf-1 kinase is essential for eosinophil activation and degranulation. J Exp Med. 1998;188:421–9.
31. Adachi T, Alam R. The mechanism of IL-5 signal transduction. Am J Physiol. 1998;275:C623–33.
32. Takatsu K, Nakajima H. IL-5 and eosinophilia. Curr Opin Immunol. 2008;20:288–94.
33. Bates ME, Green VL, Bertics PJ. ERK1 and ERK2 activation by chemotactic factors in human eosinophils is interleukin 5-dependent and contributes to leukotriene C4 biosynthesis. J Biol Chem. 2000;275:10968–75.
34. Pelaia G, Cuda G, Vatrella A, et al. Mitogen-activated protein kinases and asthma. J Cell Physiol. 2005;202:642–53.
35. Adachi T, Choudhuri BK, Stafford S, et al. The differential role of extracellular signal-regulated kinases and p38 mitogen-activated protein kinase in eosinophil functions. J Immunol. 2000;165:2198–204.
36. Ip WK, Wong CK, Wang CB, et al. Interleukin-3, −5, and granulocyte macrophage colony-stimulating factor induce adhesion and chemotaxis of human eosinophils via p38 mitogen-activated protein kinase and nuclear factor-kB. Immunopharmacol Immunotoxicol. 2005;27:371–93.
37. Sano M, Leff AR, Myou S, et al. Regulation of interleukin-5-induced β2-integrin adhesion of human eosinophils by phosphoinositide 3-kinase. Am J Respir Cell Mol Biol. 2005;33:65–70.
38. Gallelli L, Busceti MT, Vatrella A, et al. Update on anticytokine treatment for asthma. Biomed Res Int. 2013;2013:104315.
39. Garlisi CG, Kung TT, Wang P, et al. Effects of chronic anti-interleukin-5 monoclonal antibody treatment in a murine model of pulmonary inflammation. Am J Respir Cell Mol Biol. 1999;20:248–55.
40. Mauser PJ, Pitman AM, Fernandez X, et al. Effects of an antibody to interleukin-5 in a monkey model of asthma. Am J Respir Crit Care Med. 1995;152:467–72.
41. Pelaia G, Vatrella A, Maselli R. The potential of biologics for the treatment of asthma. Nat Rev Drug Discov. 2012;11:958–72.
42. Walsh GM. Therapeutic potential of targeting interleukin-5 in asthma. BioDrugs. 2013;27:559–63.
43. Patterson MF, Borish L, Kennedy JL. The past, present, and future of monoclonal antibodies to IL-5 and eosinophilic asthma. J Asthma Allergy. 2015;8:125–34.
44. Gnanakumaran G, Babu KS. Technology evaluation: mepolizumab GlaxoSmithKline. Curr Opin Mol Ther. 2003;5:321–5.
45. Walsh GM. Mepolizumab-based therapy in asthma: an update. Curr Opin Allergy Clin Immunol. 2015;15:392–6.
46. Fainardi V, Pisi G, Chetta A. Mepolizumab in the treatment of severe eosinophilic asthma. Immunotherapy. 2016;8:27–34.
47. Hart TK, Cook RM, Zia-Amirhosseini P, et al. Preclinical efficacy and safety of mepolizumab (SB-240563), a humanized monoclonal antibody to IL-5, in cynomolgus monkeys. J Allergy Clin Immunol. 2001;108:250–7.

48. Leckie MJ, ten Brinke A, Khan J, et al. Effects of an interleukin-5 blocking monoclonal antibody on eosinophils, airway hyper-responsiveness, and the late asthmatic response. Lancet. 2000;356:2144–8.
49. Flood-Page P, Swenson C, Faiferman I, et al. A study to evaluate safety and efficacy of mepolizumab in patients with moderate persistent asthma. Am J Respir Crit Care Med. 2007;176:1062–71.
50. Buttner C, Lun A, Splettstoesser T, et al. Monoclonal anti-interleukin-5 treatment suppresses eosinophil but not T-cell functions. Eur Respir J. 2003;21:799–803.
51. Haldar P, Brightling CE, Hargadon B, et al. Mepolizumab and exacerbations of refractory eosinophilic asthma. N Engl J Med. 2009;360:973–84.
52. Nair P, Pizzichini MM, Kjarsgaard M, et al. Mepolizumab for prednisone-dependent asthma with sputum eosinophilia. N Engl J Med. 2009;360:985–93.
53. Flood-Page P, Menzies-Gow A, Phipps S, et al. Anti-IL-5 treatment reduces deposition of ECM proteins in the bronchial subepithelial basement membrane of mild atopic asthmatics. J Clin Invest. 2003;112:1029–36.
54. Makinde T, Murphy RF, Agrawall DK. The regulatory role of TGF-β in airway remodeling in asthma. Immunol Cell Biol. 2007;85:348–56.
55. Pavord ID, Korn S, Howarth P, et al. Mepolizumab for severe eosinophilic asthma (DREAM): a multicentre, double-blind, placebo-controlled trial. Lancet. 2012;380:651–9.
56. Liu Y, Zhang S, Li DW, Jiang SJ. Efficacy of antiinterleukin-5 therapy with mepolizumab in patients with asthma: a meta-analysis of randomized placebo-controlled trials. PLoS One. 2013;8:e59872.
57. Bel EH, Wenzel SE, Thompson PJ, et al.; SIRIUS investigators. Oral glucocorticoid-sparing effect of mepolizumab in eosinophilic asthma. N Engl J Med. 2014;371:1189–97.
58. Ortega HG, Liu MC, Pavord ID, et al.; MENSA Investigators. Mepolizumab treatment in patients with severe eosinophilic asthma. N Engl J Med. 2014;371:1198–207.
59. Magnan A, Bourdin A, Prazma CM, et al. Treatment response with mepolizumab in severe eosinophilic asthma patients with previous omalizumab treatment. Allergy. 2016; 71:1335.
60. Menzella F, Lusuardi M, Galeone C, et al. Profile of anti-IL-5 mAb mepolizumab in the treatment of severe refractory asthma and hypereosinophilic disorders. J Asthma Allergy. 2015;8:105–14.
61. Nair P. Anti-interleukin-5 monoclonal antibody to treat severe eosinophilic asthma. N Engl J Med. 2014;371:1249–51.
62. Roufosse FE, Kahn JE, Gleich GJ, et al. Long-term safety of mepolizumab for the treatment of hypereosinophilic syndromes. J Allergy Clin Immunol. 2013;131:461–7.
63. Global Initiative for Asthma (GINA). Global strategy for asthma management and prevention. Available from: http://www.ginasthma.org.
64. Chung KF. Targeting the interleukin pathway in the treatment of asthma. Lancet. 2015;386:1086–96.
65. Walsh GM. Profile of reslizumab in eosinophilic disease and its potential in the treatment of poorly controlled eosinophilic asthma. Biologics. 2013;7:7–11.
66. Egan RW, Athwal D, Bodmer MW, et al. Effect of Sch 55700, a humanized monoclonal antibody to human interleukin-5, on eosinophilic responses and bronchial hyperreactivity. Arzneimittelforschung. 1999;49:779–90.
67. Cardet JC, Israel E. Update on reslizumab for eosinophilic asthma. Expert Opin Biol Ther. 2015;15:1531–9.
68. Lim H, Nair P. Efficacy and safety of reslizumab in patients with moderate to severe eosinophilic asthma. Expert Rev Respir Med. 2015;9:135–42.
69. Zhang J, Kuvelkar R, Murgolo NJ, et al. Mapping and characterization of the epitope(s) of Sch 55700, a humanized mAb, that inhibits human IL-5. Int Immunol. 1999;11:1935–44.
70. Kips JC, O'Connor BJ, Langley SJ, et al. Effects of SCH55700, a humanized anti-human interleukin-5 antibody, in severe persistent asthma: a pilot study. Am J Respir Crit Care Med. 2003;167:1655–9.

71. Castro M, Mathur S, Hargreave F, et al. Reslizumab for poorly controlled, eosinophilic asthma: a randomized, placebo-controlled study. Am J Respir Crit Care Med. 2011;184:1125–32.
72. Castro M, Zangrilli J, Wechsler ME, et al. Reslizumab for inadequately controlled asthma with elevated blood eosinophil counts: results from two multicentre, parallel, double-blind, randomised, placebo-controlled, phase 3 trials. Lancet Respir Med. 2015;3:355–66.
73. Bjermer L, Lemiere C, Maspero J, et al. Reslizumab for inadequately controlled asthma with elevated blood eosinophil levels: a randomized phase 3 study. Chest. 2016;3692:47551.
74. Corren J, Weinstein S, Janka L, et al. Phase 3 study of reslizumab in patients with poorly controlled asthma: effects across a broad range of eosinophil counts. Chest 2016; 150:799–810.
75. Koike M, Nakamura K, Futuya A, et al. Establishment of humanized anti-interelukin-5 receptor α chain monoclonal antibodies having a potent neutralizing activity. Hum Antibodies. 2009;18:17–27.
76. Ghazi A, Trikha A, Calhoun WJ. Benralizumab – a humanized mAb to IL-5Rα with enhanced antibody-dependent cell-mediated cytotoxicity – a novel approach for the treatment of asthma. Expert Opin Biol Ther. 2012;12:113–8.
77. Shields RL, Lai J, Keck R, et al. Lack of fucose on human IgG1 N-linked oligosaccharide improves binding to FcγRIII and antibody-dependent cellular toxicity. J Biol Chem. 2002;277:26733–40.
78. Shinkawa T, Nakamura K, Yamane N, et al. The absence of fucose but not the presence of galactose or bisecting N-acetylglucosamine of human IgG1 complex-type oligosaccharide shows the critical role of enhancing antibody-dependent cellular cytotoxicity. J Biol Chem. 2003;278:3466–73.
79. Kolbeck R, Kozhich A, Koike M, et al. Medi-563, a humanized anti-IL-5 receptor α mAb with enhanced antibody-dependent cell mediated cytotoxicity function. J Allergy Clin Immunol. 2010;125:1344–53.
80. Busse WW, Katial R, Gossage D, et al. Safety profile, pharmacokinetics, and biologic activity of MEDI-563, an anti-IL-5 receptor α antibody, in a phase I study of subjects with mild asthma. J Allergy Clin Immunol. 2010;125:1237–44.
81. Laviolette M, Gossage DL, Gauvreau G, et al. Effects of benralizumab on airway eosinophils in asthmatic patients with sputum eosinophilia. J Allergy Clin Immunol. 2013;132:1086–96.
82. Assa'ad A, Rothenberg ME. Eosinophilic asthma: insights into the effects of IL-5 receptor targeting. J Allergy Clin Immunol. 2013;132:1086–96.
83. Park HS, Kim MK, Imai N, et al. A phase 2a study of benralizumab for patients with eosinophilic asthma in South Korea and Japan. Int Arch Allergy Immunol. 2016;169:135–45.
84. Castro M, Wenzel SE, Bleecker ER. Benralizumab, an anti-interleukin 5 receptor α monoclonal antibody, versus placebo for uncontrolled eosinophilic asthma: a phase 2b randomized dose-ranging study. Lancet Respir Med. 2014;2:878–90.
85. Nowak RM, Parker JM, Silverman RA. A randomized trial of benralizumab, an antiinterleukin 5 receptor α monoclonal antibody, after acute asthma. Am J Emerg Med. 2015;33:14–20.
86. Varricchi G, Bagnasco D, Borriello F, et al. Interleukin-5 pathway inhibition in the treatment of eosinophilic respiratory disorders: evidence and unmet needs. Curr Opin Allergy Clin Immunol. 2016;16:186–200.
87. Wagener AH, de Nijs SB, Lutter R. External validation of blood eosinophils, FE(NO) and serum periostin as surrogates for sputum eosinophils in asthma. Thorax. 2015;70:115–20.
88. Pavord ID, Agusti A. Blood eosinophil count: a biomarker of an important treatable trait in patients with airway disease. Eur Respir J. 2016;47:1299–303.
89. George L, Brightling CE. Eosinophilic airway inflammation: role in asthma and chronic obstructive pulmonary disease. Ther Adv Chronic Dis. 2016;7:34–51.

Anti-IL-4/IL-13 Biologics

6

The recent advances in our understanding of asthma pathobiology can have relevant implications in both present and future therapeutic approaches. Within this context, the current more detailed knowledge of the key cellular and molecular mechanisms underlying asthma is unravelling potential targets such as IL-4 and IL-13 for the development and implementation of new biological therapies [1].

Role of IL-4 and IL-13 in Asthma Pathobiology

IL-4 and IL-13 are mainly secreted by $CD4^+$ Th2 and group 2 innate lymphoid cells (ILC2s) and also produced in lower quantities by mast cells, eosinophils, basophils, $CD8^+$ Th cells and natural killer cells [2, 3]. These cytokines are noticeably implicated in many aspects of both inflammatory and structural changes characterizing asthmatic airways (Fig. 6.1). Indeed, at the level of B lymphocytes, IL-4 and IL-13 drive Ig class switching from either IgM or IgG antibodies to IgE [5]. Furthermore, these cytokines enhance airway smooth muscle (ASM) contractility and induce airway recruitment of eosinophils by eliciting eotaxin synthesis and up-regulation of endothelial adhesion molecules such as vascular cell adhesion molecule (VCAM-1). IL-13 also stimulates mucus production and airway epithelial cell expression of inducible nitric oxide (NO) synthase. Moreover, IL-13 significantly promotes airway remodelling in asthma by enhancing goblet cell hyperplasia, transformation of bronchial fibroblasts into myofibroblasts, deposition of collagen and proliferation of airway smooth muscle (ASM) cells (Fig. 6.1) [3]. All these pro-inflammatory and structural changes induced by IL-4 and IL-13 lead to a remarkable increase in bronchial hyperresponsiveness.

When compared with non-asthmatic controls, subjects with asthma can exhibit high IL-13 levels in peripheral blood, induced sputum, bronchoalveolar lavage fluid (BALF) and bronchial mucosa [6–8]. Indeed, asthmatic patients undergoing segmental allergen challenges experience significant airway increases of both IL-13 mRNA and protein levels [9]. Furthermore, genetic research has also detected relevant linkages of IL-13/IL-13 receptor gene polymorphisms with asthma prevalence and bronchial hyperresponsiveness [10]. Thus, genetic control of IL-13 contributes to individual susceptibility to asthma, which is associated with multiple polymorphisms found in the RAD50-IL-13 region of chromosome 5q31.1 [11]. Although the effects of IL-13 largely duplicate and overlap those of IL-4, it can be argued that

© Springer International Publishing Switzerland 2017
G. Pelaia et al., *Asthma: Targeted Biological Therapies*,
DOI 10.1007/978-3-319-46007-9_6

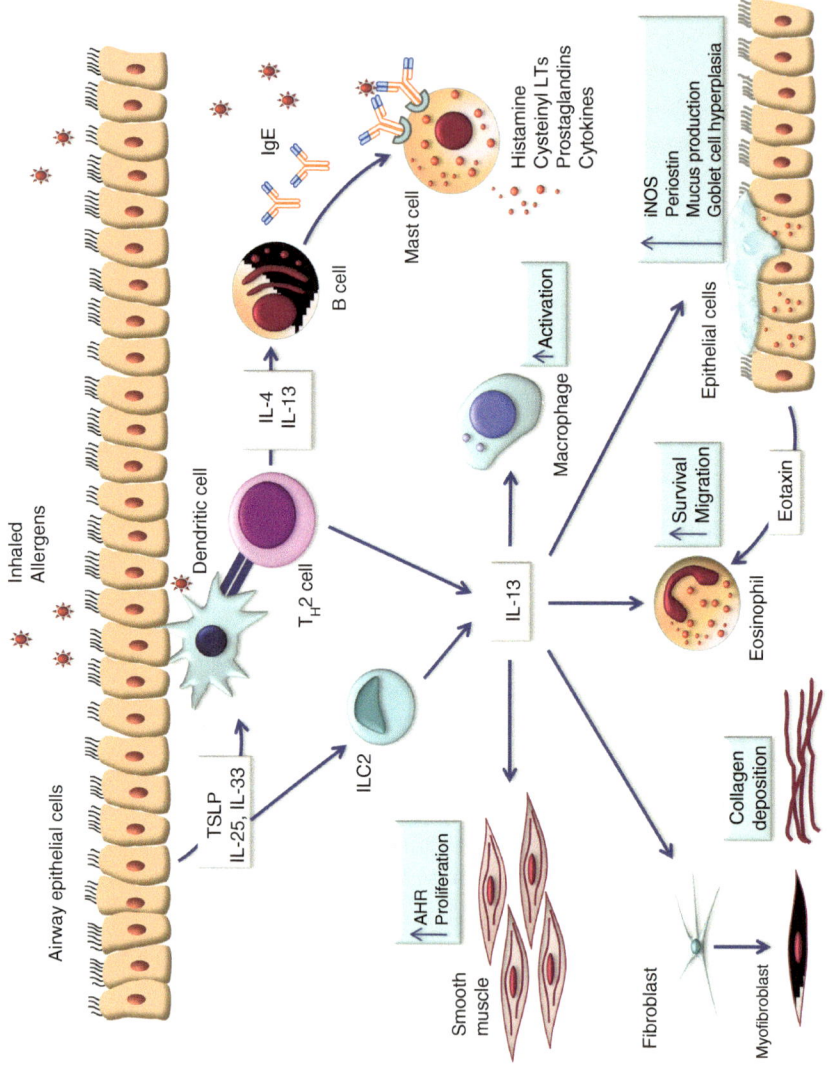

Fig. 6.1 Pleiotropic effects of IL-4 and IL-13 in asthma pathobiology. See text for details (Reprinted from Ref. [4])

these apparently very similar cytokines, also sharing common receptor mechanisms and signal transduction pathways, exert distinct biological roles in asthma. In fact, IL-4 primarily and uniquely triggers the initial commitment of naïve CD4$^+$ Th cells to a Th2 phenotype, whereas IL-13 is probably more important than IL-4 in inducing bronchial hyperresponsiveness by enhancing airway inflammation and structural changes, including subepithelial fibrosis and increased ASM thickness (Fig. 6.1) [12, 13]. These considerations are corroborated by the detection of higher concentrations of IL-13, with respect to IL-4, in murine lungs sensitized to allergens as well as in the airways of asthmatic patients, where IL-13-synthesizing cells significantly outnumber those producing IL-4 [14, 15]. Therefore, the likely differential roles of IL-4 and IL-13 in asthma pathobiology make this latter cytokine a more suitable target than IL-4 for biological antiasthma therapies.

IL-4 and IL-13 play their biological roles by activating a heterodimeric receptor complex consisting of the IL-4 receptor α-subunit (IL-4Rα) and the IL-13 receptor α1-subunit (IL-13Rα1) [16] (Fig. 6.2), which are expressed on B lymphocytes, dendritic cells, monocytes/macrophages, eosinophils, basophils, endothelial cells, bronchial epithelial cells, fibroblasts and ASM cells. Overall, the interactions of IL-4 and IL-13 with the IL-4Rα/IL-13Rα1 transmembrane complex induce the stimulation of tyrosine kinase protein Janus kinase 1/Janus kinase 2 (JAK1/JAK2) and tyrosine kinase 2 (Tyk2) [17, 18], which are situated within the cytoplasm and are constitutively associated with IL-4/IL-13 receptor chains (Fig. 6.2). Activation of these two signalling enzymes is responsible for the subsequent phosphorylation-dependent stimulation and nuclear translocation of signal transducer and activator of transcription 6 (STAT-6) [17, 18] (Fig. 6.2), which is a transcription factor that coordinates the expression of several target genes. The latter encode many molecules that act as key mediators of the biological effects of IL-4 and IL-13. The mechanism of action of IL-13 can be inhibited by its binding to IL-13 receptor α2-chain (IL-13Rα2), which does not interact with any other receptor subunit or signalling pathway (Fig. 6.2), thereby mediating an endogenous auto-regulatory negative loop that limits IL-13 activity [19].

IL-4-/IL-13-Targeted Therapies

Given the very important roles played by IL-4 and IL-13 in asthma pathobiology, several biologic drugs have been developed with the aim of inhibiting the pathophysiologic actions exerted by either IL-4, IL-13 or both cytokines in asthmatic patients.

Pascolizumab

Pascolizumab (SB 240683) is an anti-IL-4 humanized monoclonal antibody, generated by grafting complementarity-determining regions from the parental murine antihuman IL-4 antibody (3B9) into human IgG1 kappa heavy- and light-chain

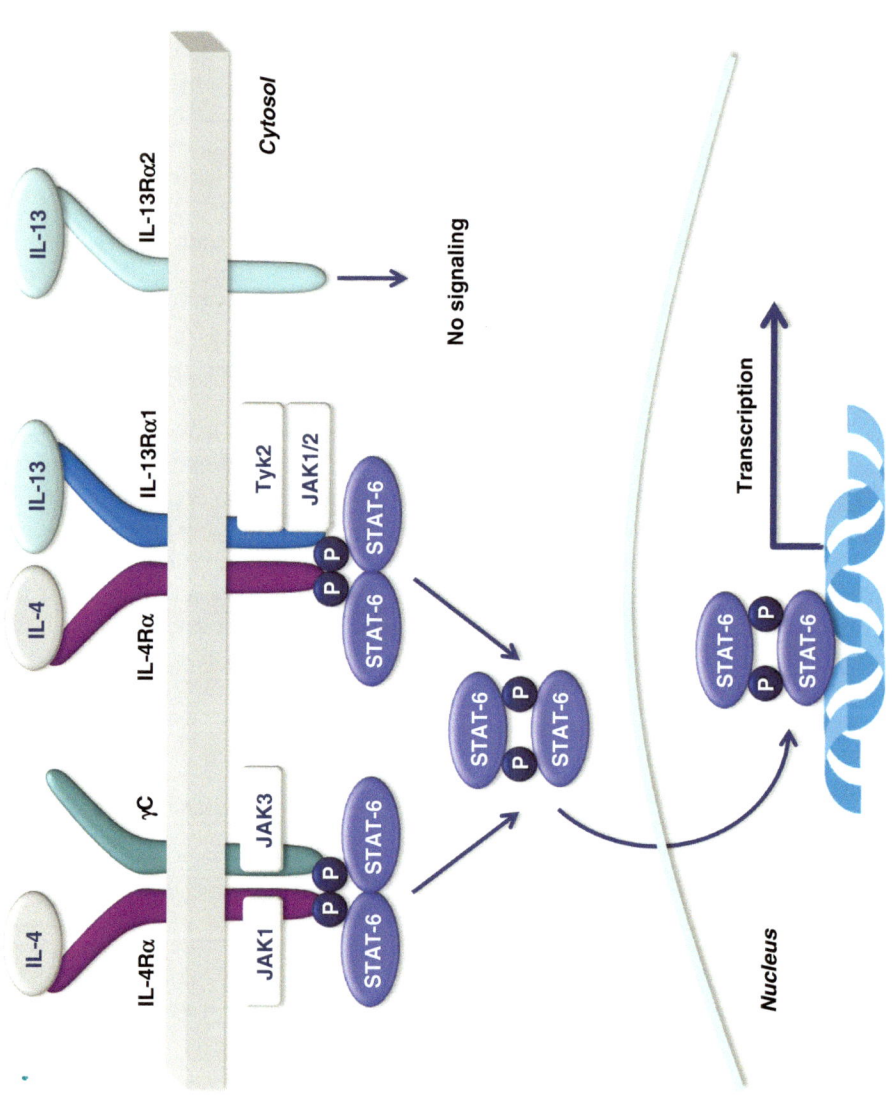

Fig. 6.2 Membrane receptors and intracellular signalling pathways activated by IL-4/IL-13. IL-4 and IL-13 exert their biological actions by activating a heterodimeric receptor complex consisting of the IL-4 receptor α-subunit (IL-4Rα) and the IL-13 receptor α1-subunit (IL-13Rα1). Binding of IL-13 to IL-13Rα1 induces heterodimerization with IL-4Rα. This dimerization, which can also be triggered by IL-4, activates JAK1/JAK2 and Tyk2 tyrosine kinases that are responsible for phosphorylation of STAT-6. Phosphorylated STAT-6 dimerizes and migrates from cytosol to the nucleus, where it binds to the promoter regions of IL-4-/IL-13-responsive genes. IL-13 can also bind to its receptor α2-chain (IL-13Rα2) that is not coupled to any dimerization mechanism or intracellular signalling pathway. The receptor/signalling complex constituted by IL-4Rα and γC chain, associated with JAK1/JAK3 kinases, can be activated only by IL-4, but not by IL-13 (Reprinted from Ref. [4])

frameworks [20]. Therefore, pascolizumab prevents IL-4 from binding to the IL-4Rα subunit. In vitro, pascolizumab effectively blocked the proliferation of T and B cells and also suppressed IL-4-dependent synthesis of IgE. Moreover, pascolizumab displayed a good tolerability profile in cynomolgus monkeys receiving up to 100 mg/kg intravenous doses every month for 9 months [20]. This positive safety pattern was confirmed by a phase 1, dose-rising study performed in subjects with mild-to-moderate asthma, who were monitored for 55 days after administration of a single intravenous dose of pascolizumab ranging from 0.5 to 10 mg/kg [21]. However, a further larger multidose, phase 2 trial was interrupted because pascolizumab did not produce any clinical benefit in patients with symptomatic, steroid-naïve asthma [21].

Pitrakinra

A better therapeutic profile than pascolizumab was shown by pitrakinra [22]. Differently from pascolizumab, pitrakinra is not an anti-IL-4 antibody but a mutein obtained by site-directed changes performed on IL-4 amino-acid sequence [23]. In particular, the arginine and tyrosine residues located at positions 121 and 124, respectively, were substituted by aspartic acid molecules. As a result of this mutagenic bioengineering technology, a ligand was generated which binds with high affinity to the IL-4Rα chain, but does not trigger downstream signalling, thereby behaving as a dual IL-4/IL-13 antagonist [24]. When received subcutaneously or via inhalation by asthmatic patients, pitrakinra was well tolerated, attenuated both early and late allergic bronchoconstrictive reactions and also decreased exacerbations of eosinophilic asthma [25, 26]. Furthermore, in a pharmacogenetic, placebo-controlled trial focused on modulation of IL-4-/IL-13-mediated actions, several doses (1, 3 or 10 mg twice a day for 12 weeks) of inhaled pitrakinra were evaluated in asthmatic patients with moderate-to-severe disease [27]. This study showed that pitrakinra, though not being clinically effective in the entire population of recruited subjects, at the dosage of 10 mg, significantly reduced asthma exacerbation rates in patients exhibiting specific single-nucleotide polymorphisms in the 3′ untranslated region of the IL-4Rα gene (rs8832GG and rs1029489GG genotypes) [27].

Dupilumab

Another combined therapeutic approach targeting both IL-4 and IL-13 has been realized by developing dupilumab, a fully human monoclonal antibody directed against IL-4Rα subunit [4]. Therefore, dupilumab is capable of blocking the signal transduction pathways activated by IL-4 and IL-13.

The therapeutic effects of dupilumab were evaluated in asthmatic individuals with persistent, moderate-to-severe disease and airway or peripheral eosinophilia [28]. In particular, 104 subjects aged from 18 to 65 years were recruited, who had a mean baseline forced expiratory volume in 1 s (FEV_1) calculated as 72 % of predicted value, as well as at least 300 eosinophils per microlitre of peripheral blood or at least 3 % eosinophils in induced sputum. They used long-acting β_2-adrenergic agonists (LABAs) added to medium/high inhaled corticosteroid (ICS) doses, without achieving a satisfactory asthma control. Fifty-two patients were assigned to a weekly, subcutaneous treatment with dupilumab (300 mg), and 52 patients received placebo. Dupilumab was administered for 12 weeks or until patients experienced an asthma exacerbation. In addition, study patients were instructed to interrupt LABA administration after 4 weeks and to progressively reduce and then suspend their ICS therapy between weeks 6 and 9. The primary investigational outcome was the onset of an asthma exacerbation. In this regard, three patients undergoing treatment with dupilumab (6 %) experienced a disease exacerbation versus 23 subjects belonging to the placebo group (44 %). Such results correspond to an overall 87 % reduction in exacerbation rate ($P < 0.001$) in the dupilumab group. In terms of secondary end points, dupilumab induced a marked FEV_1 improvement, exceeding 200 mL, and also elicited a parallel increase in morning peak expiratory flow (PEF), associated with a smaller rise in evening PEF. Furthermore, dupilumab progressively improved the Asthma Control Questionnaire (ACQ) score throughout the study and also decreased asthmatic symptoms occurring during morning and evening, nocturnal awakenings due to asthma and use of the short-acting β_2-adrenergic agonist salbutamol as rescue medication. Dupilumab was also able to significantly ($P < 0.001$) reduce the levels of Th2-associated inflammatory biomarkers such as fractional exhaled nitric oxide (FeNO) concentrations, which were found to be markedly lower after 4 weeks of treatment and persisted up to week 12 at lesser levels than baseline values, in spite of ICS interruption. FeNO decrease was correlated to FEV_1 improvement. Similar reductions were also found in serum levels of IgE, eotaxin-3 and thymus- and activation-regulated chemokine (TARC). Conversely, no apparent changes in blood eosinophil counts were detected in patients treated with dupilumab. Taken together, these study findings suggest that targeting Th2-driven, uncontrolled asthma with a therapeutic strategy aimed to neutralize the biological effects of both IL-4 and IL-13 at the receptor level can be more effective than blocking the actions of IL-4 alone. Because about 80 % of the enrolled patients used high ICS doses, it can be argued that dupilumab may be successful in inhibiting residual and relatively ICS/LABA-refractory airway inflammation, mainly sustained by IL-4 and IL-13 in subjects with poorly controlled asthma. However, despite the evident benefits manifested by asthmatic patients undergoing treatment with dupilumab, relevant criticisms can be raised to this trial [4, 29]. Firstly, on the basis of such a study, it is not possible to understand whether dupilumab can be also effective in other asthmatic populations, like those not exhibiting Th2-mediated airway and/or blood eosinophilia. Secondly, an obvious weakness of this trial is strictly intrinsic to its design, based on an unusual ICS/LABA withdrawal, which is very unlikely to occur in clinical practice. Indeed, this feature of the experimental protocol precluded the possibility of evaluating the potential additive value of dupilumab with regard to the standard controller therapy of asthma, commonly represented by ICS/LABA associations. On the other hand, in real life physicians do not withdraw ICS and LABAs in patients with difficult-to-control asthma. For instance, during the first part of the study, when all enrolled subjects were taking ICS and LABAs, no meaningful change in exacerbation rate was found in the dupilumab group, when compared with the placebo arm. At the same early time points, only very mild improvements in lung function and inflammatory biomarkers were observed in patients receiving dupilumab. Finally, when considering the safety and tolerability profile with respect to placebo, a higher frequency of injection-site reactions, nasopharyngitis, nausea and headache was reported during treatment with dupilumab. Moreover, progressive cutaneous rush, urticaria and oedema occurred in one patient receiving dupilumab, requiring non-urgent symptomatic therapy (systemic corticosteroids and antihistamine drugs) and immediate interruption of study treatment. Intriguingly and unexpectedly, dupilumab apparently increased eosinophil levels in four patients. Therefore, given the limited size of the study population ($n = 52$) treated with dupilumab in this trial, the overall range of possible unwanted reactions is largely not known, and close monitoring for such adverse events is thus necessary.

A larger, phase 2b dose-ranging study has been recently carried out in adult patients with uncontrolled persistent asthma, despite the use of medium-to-high doses of ICS/LABA, which were not discontinued during the add-on therapy with dupilumab [30]. The trial consisted of three periods including a 14–21-day screening period, a 24-week randomized treatment period and a 16-week posttreatment follow-up period. 776 subjects were randomly subdivided into five groups, assigned to receive subcutaneous injections of placebo ($n = 158$), dupilumab at doses of 200 mg every 2 weeks ($n = 150$) or 4 weeks ($n = 154$) or dupilumab at doses of 300 mg every 2 weeks ($n = 157$) or 4 weeks ($n = 157$), respectively. With the exception of the group receiving the dosage of 200 mg every 4 weeks, in comparison to placebo, all dupilumab dose regimens elicited significant FEV_1 increases, ranging at week 24 from 0.15 to 0.16 L. Furthermore, when given every 2 weeks and compared with placebo, dupilumab significantly decreased the annualized rates of severe asthma exacerbations. All dupilumab dosage regimens also induced significant dose-dependent decreases in FeNO, which were greater when the drug was administered every 2 weeks. With regard to the effects referring to lung function, asthma exacerbations and FeNO levels, no significant differences were detected among patients having at least 300 or less eosinophils per microlitre of peripheral blood. Overall, the reported adverse events were similar across the five study arms and mainly included upper respiratory tract infections, injection-site erythema and headache. Transient increases of blood eosinophils were found in patients with baseline eosinophil counts of at least 300 cells per microlitre of blood. Therefore, this important trial showed that dupilumab is well tolerated and provides relevant clinical, functional and anti-inflammatory effects in adult patients with uncontrolled persistent asthma, regardless of their blood eosinophil numbers. Because dupilumab resulted to be more effective when administered every 2 weeks, this interval between subcutaneous injections has been chosen to further evaluate drug efficacy in an ongoing phase 3 clinical trial (NCT02414854).

Anti-IL-4/IL-13 Bispecific Antibodies

A further strategy aimed to generate biologic drugs capable of suppressing the bio-activity of IL-4 and IL-13 is based on the development of human bispecific antibodies targeting both these cytokines. Differently from monoclonal antibodies, which are selectively directed against a single antigen, bispecific antibodies can simultaneously target two diverse antigens. In this regard, anti-IL-4/IL-13 IgG1 and IgG4 antibodies have been constructed, which retain the high affinities and binding properties of the parental Fab(s) towards IL-4 and IL-13 epitopes, thereby displaying powerful IL-4/IL-13 neutralizing actions in in vitro cellular assays [31]. Moreover, pharmacokinetic studies performed in cynomolgus monkeys showed that after intravenous administration, these IgG1 and IgG4 bispecific antibodies partitioned comparably from serum to the lungs, thus reaching relatively high levels in the airways, where they can effectively counteract the pathogenic activity of IL-4 and IL-13 [32]. Hence, this therapeutic approach appears to be very promising for the treatment of asthma.

Lebrikizumab

Lebrikizumab is an IgG4 humanized monoclonal antibody which binds with very high affinity to IL-13, thereby inhibiting its interaction with the IL-4/IL-13 receptor complex and abrogating IL-13 functions [32, 33]. In particular, lebrikizumab can inhibit IL-13-dependent STAT6 phosphorylation and cell proliferation in TF-1 cells (human erythroleukemic cell line) [33]. In this regard, it has been shown that lebrikizumab exerted significant therapeutic actions in Th2-mediated asthma, which can also be identified by the detection of high serum levels of periostin [34]. Encoded by an IL-13-inducible gene, periostin is a matricellular protein produced by inflammatory cells, bronchial epithelium and lung fibroblasts, which is involved in many aspects of asthma pathobiology such as eosinophil recruitment, enhanced expression of pro-inflammatory mediators and airway remodelling [35–37]. Periostin is secreted into the extracellular matrix from the basolateral surface of airway epithelial cells stimulated with IL-13 and then accumulates in bronchial circulation and peripheral bloodstream, thus being considered as a systemic marker of eosinophilic asthma [37].

A phase 2 placebo-controlled trial performed by Corren et al. demonstrated that lebrikizumab, when added to guideline-based antiasthma inhaled treatment, is very well tolerated [38]. This 6-month study, involving 219 adult asthmatic subjects not adequately controlled by inhaled corticosteroids, evaluated the therapeutic activity of lebrikizumab given by the subcutaneous route every month at a dose of 250 mg. Lebrikizumab elicited its best effects in moderate-to-severe asthmatic patients with high blood concentrations of periostin. Indeed, significant FEV_1 improvements, resulting in a 5.5 % increase with respect to baseline levels, were found in the whole population of enrolled patients after 12 weeks of treatment with lebrikizumab. In particular, FEV_1 increased by 8.2 % in the group of patients with high levels of periostin and by 1.6 % (not significant) in the group of patients with low periostin concentrations, respectively. Therefore, these findings suggest that periostin can be reliably utilized in real life as a biomarker of IL-13-induced asthma, which is potentially susceptible to anti-IL-13 therapeutic approaches. In the same trial, a post-lebrikizumab FEV_1 increase (8.6 %) similar to that observed in individuals exhibiting high blood levels of periostin was also found in subjects who displayed high pretreatment values of FeNO [38], another biomarker whose biosynthesis can be induced by IL-13. Indeed, lebrikizumab caused a 19 % mean reduction in FeNO after 12 weeks of treatment, which resulted to be significantly different ($P < 0.001$) versus the 10 % increase detected in patients receiving placebo. Lebrikizumab did not elicit significant changes in secondary end points including morning PEF, ACQ score, use of rescue medications and rate of asthma exacerbations. However, a report referring to a further analysis of this study stated that lebrikizumab was able to reduce severe asthma exacerbations over 32 weeks [39]. In fact, during this period the rate of severe exacerbations decreased by 50 % in the lebrikizumab group, when compared to the placebo arm ($P < 0.05$). A trend towards a greater decrease in severe exacerbation rate was detected in patients with high baseline serum levels of periostin.

In another phase 2 trial carried out by Noonan et al. in 212 asthmatic patients not receiving ICS, randomized to undergo therapy with either placebo or three different subcutaneous monthly doses (125, 250 or 500 mg for 12 weeks) of lebrikizumab, this drug induced a slight increase in mean FEV_1, which did not result to be statistically or clinically significant [40]. Moreover, with regard to patient subgroups distinguished on the basis of serum periostin concentrations, after 12 weeks of treatment, no meaningful differences in FEV_1 changes were detected between the three lebrikizumab dose groups and the placebo arm. However, the well-tolerated lebrikizumab therapy was associated with a decreased risk of treatment failure at all doses versus placebo, thereby suggesting that IL-13 blockade was capable of improving asthma control. Lebrikizumab also lowered FeNO levels.

A further phase 2 clinical investigation, conducted by Scheerens et al., evaluated the protective effect of lebrikizumab in patients with mild atopic asthma undergoing whole lung challenge with inhaled aeroallergens [41]. Although this study involved only 29 patients, it led to very interesting results and conclusions. In particular, when compared to placebo, the well-tolerated subcutaneous administration of lebrikizumab (5 mg/Kg every 4 weeks for 12 weeks) produced a 48 % decrease in the late asthmatic response, though this effect did not result to be statistically significant. However, a further subgroup analysis showed that, when compared to subjects with relatively low baseline levels of serum IgE, peripheral blood eosinophils and serum periostin, a greater reduction in the late asthmatic response was exhibited by patients carrying high concentrations of these biomarkers. In addition, lebrikizumab significantly decreased the concentrations of systemic markers of Th2 inflammation including serum IgE, as well as chemokine ligands 13 (CCL13) and 17 (CCL17) [41].

The phase 2b multicentre VERSE (258 patients) and LUTE (205 patients) replicate studies collectively evaluated 463 uncontrolled asthmatics, treated with medium-to-high doses of ICS plus a second controller medication [42]. These patients were randomly subdivided in four groups receiving either placebo or one of three different doses (37.5, 125 or 250 mg) of subcutaneous lebrikizumab, administered every 4 weeks for a median add-on treatment duration of approximately 24 weeks. In comparison to placebo, a pooled analysis of the two trials showed that lebrikizumab decreased the rate of asthma exacerbations (primary end point) by 60 % in periostin-high subjects and only by 5 % in periostin-low patients. Furthermore, in patients with high baseline blood levels of periostin, lebrikizumab increased the time to first exacerbation and reduced the need for urgent asthma-related healthcare use. In periostin-high subjects, after 12 weeks of treatment, lebrikizumab enhanced FEV_1 versus placebo by 6.8 %, 10.7 % and 10.1 % at doses of 37.5 mg, 125 mg and 250 mg, respectively. Otherwise, in periostin-low patients the mean FEV_1 changes induced by lebrikizumab versus placebo, with respect to baseline values, were -1.9 %, 2.2 % and 7.2 % at doses of 37.5 mg, 125 mg and 250 mg, respectively. Hence, the results of these two studies further corroborate the evidence supporting the role of periostin as a predictive biomarker of the therapeutic benefits achievable with lebrikizumab treatment. In addition to periostin, relatively high levels of FeNO (≥ 21 ppb) and blood eosinophils (≥ 240 cells/µl) were also predictive of positive treatment responses to lebrikizumab. With regard to safety, the incidence of adverse events was quite similar through the four groups of the two studies. Only injection-site reactions occurred more frequently during treatments with lebrikizumab at 125 and 250 mg doses, when compared with the 37.5 mg dose or placebo. Anaphylaxis, anaphylactoid events or serious hypersensitivity reactions were not reported during the two replicate studies. In order to confirm and extend all these findings, larger placebo-controlled phase 3 trials are currently underway.

Tralokinumab

Tralokinumab (CAT-354) is a fully human anti-IL-13 IgG4 antibody which markedly suppressed bronchial hyperresponsiveness and airway eosinophilia in a murine model of IL-13-induced lung inflammation [43–45]. Later tested at different doses in a double-blind, randomized and placebo-controlled phase 1 study, tralokinumab exhibited a linear pharmacokinetic profile and a satisfactory safety pattern when administered intravenously (1.5 or 10 mg/Kg) every 28 days [21]. In a placebo-controlled phase 2 study performed by Piper et al. in 194 asthmatic patients with moderate-to-severe uncontrolled disease, the effects of tralokinumab were investigated by administering this drug subcutaneously (150, 300 or 600 mg) at 2-week intervals, as add-on therapy to standard controller treatment [46]. Comparative evaluation between tralokinumab and placebo did not show any significant difference with regard to ACQ symptom score. However, tralokinumab significantly decreased the use of as-needed short-acting bronchodilators and also enhanced percentage FEV_1 values with respect to baseline levels; FEV_1 increases were included within an 8.1 % (150 mg) to 16.1 % (600 mg) range. When compared to patients with no sputum IL-13, FEV_1 increases were higher in asthmatic subjects exhibiting detectable IL-13 levels in their induced sputum. Tralokinumab was well tolerated and did not induce any serious adverse event.

In a subsequent phase 2b double-blind, multicentre study carried out by Brightling et al., 452 patients with severe uncontrolled asthma who had at least two, but no more than six, exacerbations during the previous 12 months were randomly assigned to receive either placebo ($n = 151$) or 300 mg of subcutaneous tralokinumab every 2 weeks ($n = 150$) or every 4 weeks ($n = 151$) [47]. Among the 383 subjects who completed the study up to week 52, the annual rates of asthma exacerbations were not significantly different between patients treated with tralokinumab and those receiving placebo. Differences in asthma exacerbation rates did not reach the threshold of statistical significance even when patients were stratified on the basis of their serum levels of potential biomarkers of IL-13 pathway activation such as periostin or dipeptidyl peptidase-4 (DPP-4), a multifunctional enzyme which is overexpressed in both plasma and CD4+ T lymphocytes from subjects with asthma [48]. However, when compared with placebo, tralokinumab administered every 2 weeks, but not every 4 weeks, significantly enhanced FEV_1 values. In particular, with respect to baseline levels, FEV_1 increased by 7.28 % ($p = 0.003$) after treatment with tralokinumab every 2 weeks and only by 1.84 % (not significant) after treatment with tralokinumab every 4 weeks, respectively. At week 52, when compared with the placebo group, FEV_1 was 10.82 % ($p = 0.005$) higher than baseline in patients with high DPP-4 serum levels, whereas a not significant 3.64 % increase in FEV_1 was recorded in subjects with low DPP-4 serum levels. Furthermore, a better improvement in FEV_1 was shown in asthmatic patients with post-bronchodilator reversibility, who were not receiving a long-term treatment with oral corticosteroids. Moreover, asthma symptom control significantly improved in the high DPP-4 subgroup, but not in the low DPP-4 subgroup. No significant improvements in asthma symptom control were observed in the subgroups with either high or low serum concentrations of periostin. Tralokinumab and placebo were characterized by overlapping safety profiles. In fact, the overall incidence of adverse events was similar across the three study groups. The most frequent side effects which occurred during treatment with tralokinumab were pain, erythema and pruritus at injection site.

With regard to the investigation of the therapeutic effects of tralokinumab in uncontrolled asthma, the potential utility of markers related to IL-13 bioactivity is currently under further evaluation in larger numbers of patients enrolled in the ongoing phase 3 trials STRATOS 1 and STRATOS 2 (ClinicalTrials.gov identifiers: NCT02161757 and NCT02194699, respectively).

GSK679586

GSK679586 is a humanized IgG1 monoclonal antibody directed against an epitope known to be very important for binding of IL-13 to both IL-13Rα1 and IL-13Rα2 receptor subunits [49]. A phase 1, placebo-controlled and dose-escalation study, performed by Hodsman et al. in healthy subjects and patients with mild asthma, showed that GSK679586 was well tolerated, displayed a linear pharmacokinetics pattern and dose- and time-dependently decreased FeNO in mild intermittent asthmatics [49]. Therefore, GSK679586 was subsequently evaluated by De Boever et al. in severe asthmatic subjects, relatively resistant to high ICS doses [50]. However, when compared with the placebo group, patients receiving a well-tolerated 12-week treatment with three once-monthly intravenous infusions of GSK679586 (10 mg/kg) did not experience any significant improvement in several clinical, functional and laboratory measurements including ACQ symptom score, asthma exacerbation rate, FEV_1, serum IgE levels and blood eosinophil counts [50].

Concluding Remarks

Because IL-4 and IL-13 significantly contribute to airway inflammation and bronchial remodelling in asthma, these two cytokines are suitable targets of biological therapies aimed to improve disease control in inadequately controlled patients. However, some relatively discordant results emerging from the currently completed trials suggest that, in order to reasonably predict the individual responses to anti-IL-4/IL-13 treatments, a detailed phenotypic characterization is necessary, possibly based on reliable markers of IL-4/IL-13 bioactivities such as periostin and DPP-4. In particular, it will be important to understand if biologic drugs targeted against IL-4 and/or IL-13 can eventually only improve symptom control in difficult-to-treat asthma or also potentially play a disease-modifying role. In this regard, larger and longer studies are needed to be carried out in selectively recruited patients in order to better elucidate the future place in asthma treatment of these specific anti-cytokine therapies.

References

1. Walsh GM. Anti-IL-4/-13 based therapy in asthma. Expert Opin Emerg Drugs. 2015;20:349–52.
2. Steinke JW, Borish L. Th2 cytokines and asthma. Interleukin 4: its role in the pathogenesis of asthma, and targeting it for asthma treatment with interleukin-4 receptor antagonists. Respir Res. 2001;2:66–70.
3. Corren J. Role of interleukin-13 in asthma. Curr Allergy Asthma Rep. 2013;13:415–20.
4. Vatrella A, Fabozzi I, Calabrese C, et al. Dupilumab: a novel treatment for asthma. J Asthma Allergy. 2014;7:123–30.
5. Froidure A, Mouthuy J, Durham SR, et al. Asthma phenotypes and IgE responses. Eur Respir J. 2016;47:304–19.
6. Saha SK, Berry MA, Parker D, et al. Increased sputum and bronchial biopsy IL-13 expression in severe asthma. J Allergy Clin Immunol. 2008;121:685–91.
7. Corren J. Anti-interleukin-13 antibody therapy for asthma: one step closer. Eur Respir J. 2013;41:255–6.
8. Maes T, Joos GF, Brusselle GG. Targeting IL-4 in asthma: lost in translation? Am J Respir Cell Mol Biol. 2012;47:261–70.
9. Prieto J, Lensmar C, Roquet AI, et al. Increased interleukin-13 mRNA expression in bronchoalveolar lavage cells of atopic patients with mild asthma after repeated low-dose allergen provocations. Respir Med. 2000;94:806–14.

10. Howard TD, Koppelman GH, Xu J, et al. Gene-gene interaction in asthma: IL4RA and IL-13 in a Dutch population with asthma. Am J Hum Genet. 2002;70:230–6.
11. Li X, Howard TD, Zheng SL, et al. Genome-wide association study of asthma identifies RAD50-IL13 and HLA-DR/DQ regions. J Allergy Clin Immunol. 2010;125:328–35.
12. Wills-Karp M, Luyimbazi J, Xu X, et al. Interleukin-13: central mediator of allergic asthma. Science. 1998;282:2258–61.
13. Grunig G, Warnock M, Wakil AE, et al. Requirement for IL-13 independently of IL-4 in experimental asthma. Science. 1998;282:2261–3.
14. Munitz A, Brandt EB, Mingler M, et al. Distinct roles for IL-13 and IL-4 via IL-13 receptor α1 and the type II IL-4 receptor in asthma pathogenesis. Proc Natl Acad Sci U S A. 2008;105:7240–5.
15. Kotsimbos TC, Ernst P, Hamid QA, et al. Interleukin-13 and interleukin-4 are coexpressed in atopic asthma. Proc Assoc Am Physicians. 1996;108:368–73.
16. Oh CK, Geba GP, Molfino N. Investigational therapeutics targeting the IL-4/IL-13/STAT-6 pathway for the treatment of asthma. Eur Respir Rev. 2010;19:46–54.
17. Andrews R, Rosa L, Daines M, Khurana HG. Reconstitution of a functional human type II IL-4/IL-13 receptor in mouse B cells: demonstration of species specificity. J Immunol. 2001;166:1716–22.
18. Chiba Y, Goto K, Misawa M. Interleukin-13-induced activation of signal transducer and activator of transcription 6 is mediated by an activation of Janus kinase 1 in cultured human bronchial smooth muscle cells. Pharmacol Rep. 2012;64:454–8.
19. Zheng T, Liu W, Oh SY, et al. IL-13 receptor α2 selectively inhibits IL-13-induced responses in the murine lung. J Immunol. 2008;180:522–9.
20. Hart TK, Blackburn MN, Brigham-Burke M, et al. Preclinical efficacy and safety of pascolizumab (SB 240683): a humanized anti-interleukin-4 antibody with therapeutic potential in asthma. Clin Exp Immunol. 2002;130:93–100.
21. Pelaia G, Vatrella A, Maselli R. The potential of biologics for the treatment of asthma. Nat Rev Drug Discov. 2012;11:958–72.
22. Gallelli L, Busceti MT, Vatrella A, et al. Update on anti-cytokine treatment for asthma. Biomed Res Int. 2013;2013:104315.
23. Antoniu SA, Cojocaru I. Pitrakinra for asthma. Expert Opin Biol Ther. 2010;10:1609–15.
24. Burmeister Getz E, Fisher DM, Fuller R. Human pharmacokinetics/pharmacodynamics of an interleukin-4 and interleukin-13 dual antagonist in asthma. J Clin Pharmacol. 2009;49:1025–36.
25. Holgate ST. Pathophysiology of asthma: what has our current understanding taught us about new therapeutic approaches? J Allergy Clin Immunol. 2011;128:495–505.
26. Wenzel S, Wilbraham D, Fuller R, et al. Effect of an interleukin-4 variant on late phase asthmatic response to allergen challenge in asthmatic patients: results of two phase 2a studies. Lancet. 2007;370:1422–31.
27. Slager RE, Otulana BA, Hawkins GA, et al. IL-4 receptor polymorphisms predict reduction in asthma exacerbations during response to an anti-IL-4 receptor α antagonist. J Allergy Clin Immunol. 2012;130:516–22.
28. Wenzel S, Ford L, Pearlman D, et al. Dupilumab in persistent asthma with elevated eosinophil levels. N Engl J Med. 2013;368:2455–66.
29. Wechsler ME. Inhibiting IL-4 and IL-13 in difficult-to-control asthma. N Engl J Med. 2013;368:2511–3.
30. Wenzel S, Castro M, Corren J, et al. Dupilumab efficacy and safety in adults with uncontrolled persistent asthma despite use of medium-to-high-dose inhaled corticosteroids plus a long-acting β2 agonist: a randomised double-blind placebo-controlled pivotal phase 2b dose-ranging trial. Lancet. 2016;388:31–44.
31. Spiess C, Bevers III J, Jackman J, et al. Development of a human IgG4 bispecific antibody for dual targeting of interleukin-4 (IL-4) and interleukin-13 (IL-13) cytokines. J Biol Chem. 2013;288:26583–93.

32. Ultsch M, Bevers J, Nakamura G, et al. Structural basis of signaling blockade by anti-IL-13 antibody lebrikizumab. J Mol Biol. 2013;425:1330–9.
33. Thomson NC, Patel M, Smith AD. Lebrikizumab in the personalized management of asthma. Biol. 2012;6:329–35.
34. Maselli DJ, Keyt H, Rogers L. Profile of lebrikizumab and its potential role in the treatment of asthma. J Asthma Allergy. 2015;8:87–92.
35. Li W, Gao P, Zhi Y, et al. Periostin: its role in asthma and its potential as a diagnostic or therapeutic target. Respir Res. 2015;16:57.
36. Takayama G, Arima K, Kanaji T, et al. Periostin: a novel component of subepithelial fibrosis of bronchial asthma downstream of IL-4 and IL-13 signals. J Allergy Clin Immunol. 2006;118:98–104.
37. Jia G, Erickson RW, Choy DF, et al. Periostin is a systemic biomarker of eosinophilic airway inflammation in asthmatic patients. J Allergy Clin Immunol. 2012;130:647–54.
38. Corren J, Lemanske RF, Hanania NA, et al. Lebrikizumab treatment in adults with asthma. N Engl J Med. 2011;365:1088–98.
39. McClintock D, Corren J, Hanania NA, et al. Lebrikizumab, an anti-IL-13 monoclonal antibody, reduces severe asthma exacerbations over 32 weeks in adults with inadequately controlled asthma. Int Conf Am Thorac Soc. (May 18–23, San Francisco), Abst 813, 2012.
40. Noonan M, Korenblat P, Mosesova S, et al. Dose-ranging study of lebrikizumab in asthmatic patients not receiving inhaled steroids. J Allergy Clin Immunol. 2013;132:567–74.
41. Scheerens H, Arron JR, Zheng Y, et al. The effects of lebrikizumab in patients with mild asthma following whole lung allergen challenge. Clin Exp Allergy. 2014;44:38–46.
42. Hanania NA, Noonan M, Corren J, et al. Lebrikizumab in moderate-to-severe asthma: pooled data from two randomised placebo-controlled studies. Thorax. 2015;70:748–56.
43. Blanchard C, Mishra A, Saito-Hakei H, et al. Inhibition of human interleukin-13-induced respiratory and oesophageal inflammation by anti-human interleukin-13 antibody (CAT-354). Clin Exp Allergy. 2005;35:1096–103.
44. Walsh GM. Tralokinumab, an anti-IL-13 mAb for the potential treatment of asthma and COPD. Curr Opin Invest Drugs. 2010;11:1305–12.
45. Antohe I, Croitoru R, Antoniu S. Tralokinumab for uncontrolled asthma. Exp Opin Biol Ther. 2013;13:323–6.
46. Piper E, Brightling C, Niven R, et al. A phase II placebo-controlled study of tralokinumab in moderate-to-severe asthma. Eur Respir J. 2013;41:330–8.
47. Brightling CE, Chanez P, Leigh R, et al. Efficacy and safety of tralokinumab in patients with severe uncontrolled asthma: a randomised, double-blind, placebo-controlled, phase 2b trial. Lancet Respir Med. 2015;3:692–701.
48. Lun SW, Wong CK, Ko FW, et al. Increased expression of plasma and CD4+ T lymphocyte costimulatory molecule CD26 in adult patients with allergic asthma. J Clin Immunol. 2007;27:430–7.
49. Hodsman P, Ashman C, Cahn A, et al. A phase 1, randomized, placebo-controlled study of an anti-IL-13 monoclonal antibody in healthy subjects and mild asthmatics. Br J Clin Pharmacol. 2012;75:118–28.
50. De Boever EH, Ashman C, Cahn AP, et al. Efficacy and safety of an anti-IL-13 mAB in patients with severe asthma: a randomized trial. J Allergy Clin Immunol. 2014;133:989–96.

Tumour necrosis factor-α (TNF-α) plays a relevant role in many features of asthma pathobiology by exerting its effects on both airway inflammatory and structural cells (Fig. 7.1) [1]. This pleiotropic cytokine is produced by several cell types including Th1 lymphocytes, macrophages and mast cells and induces the recruitment of neutrophils and eosinophils into the airways via up-regulation of epithelial and endothelial adhesion molecules [2, 3]. Moreover, by enhancing TGF-β expression, TNF-α stimulates airway smooth muscle cell proliferation, as well as fibroblast growth and maturation into myofibroblasts [4–6]. Therefore, TNF-α can contribute to the development of severe asthma not only by inducing airway inflammation and hyperresponsiveness but also by promoting bronchial remodelling [7]. Indeed, TNF-α is overexpressed in the airways of patients with severe asthma and also directly stimulates airway smooth muscle contraction through changes in intracellular calcium fluxes [1].

Therefore, several biologic drugs targeting TNF-α have been evaluated for asthma treatment in both experimental animal models and clinical studies (Fig. 7.2). In a murine model of ovalbumin-induced asthma, the fully human anti-TNF-α monoclonal antibody adalimumab reduced the peribronchiolar and perivascular infiltration of inflammatory cells and also decreased airway smooth muscle hypertrophy and oedema [8]. With regard to clinical studies, conflicting results have been obtained, and serious concerns have been raised with regard to the safety of TNF-α blockade, which may cause susceptibility to the development of respiratory infections and human cancers [9–11].

Etanercept is a soluble recombinant dimer protein consisting of two human TNF-α receptors fused with the Fc domain of human IgG1. When etanercept was administered subcutaneously at a dose of 25 mg twice weekly for 12 weeks to patients with severe asthma, there was a significant improvement in ACQ score, FEV_1, PEF and bronchial hyperresponsiveness to methacholine [12]. Similar effects on asthma symptoms and lung function were observed by Berry et al. during another study carried out in patients with severe refractory asthma, who expressed high monocyte levels of TNF-α and TNF-α receptor and received 25 mg of etanercept, given subcutaneously twice weekly for 10 weeks [7]. However, in patients with moderate-to-severe persistent asthma receiving 25 mg of subcutaneous etanercept twice weekly for 12 weeks and exhibiting a good drug tolerability, no significant differences between etanercept and placebo were later reported by Holgate et al. during a larger trial with regard to lung function, airway hyperresponsiveness,

© Springer International Publishing Switzerland 2017   83
G. Pelaia et al., *Asthma: Targeted Biological Therapies*,
DOI 10.1007/978-3-319-46007-9_7

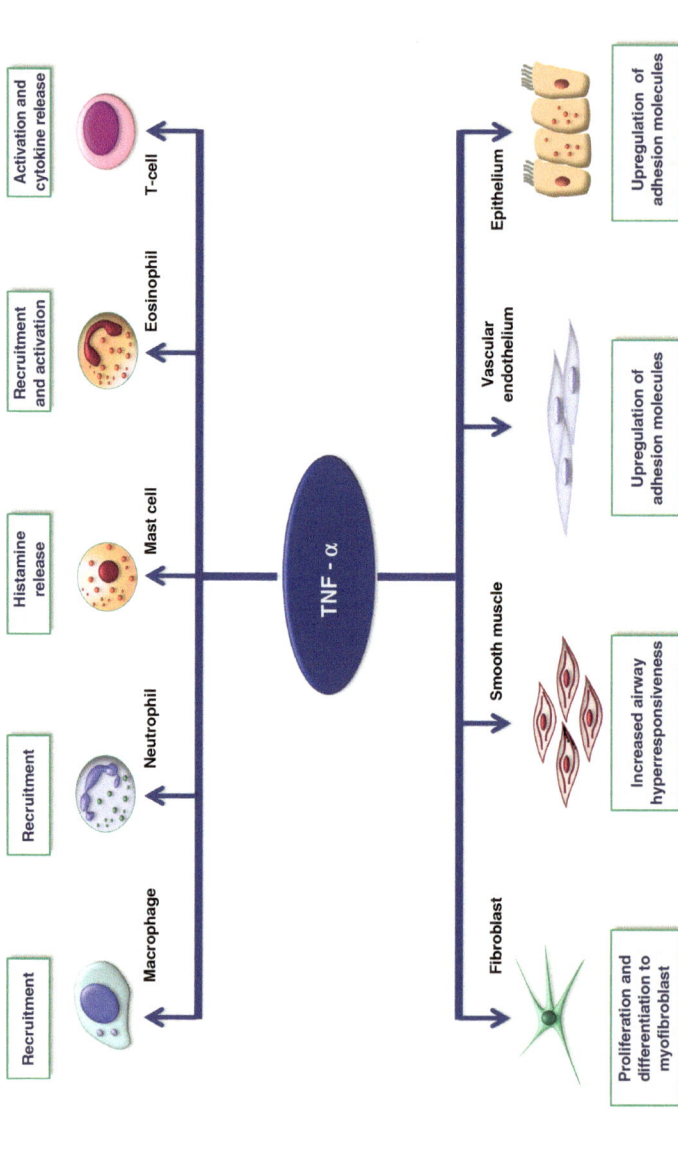

Fig. 7.1 Role of TNF-α in asthma pathobiology. In asthmatic airways, TNF-α remarkably affects the functions of both inflammatory and structural cells. See text for details (Modified from Ref. [1])

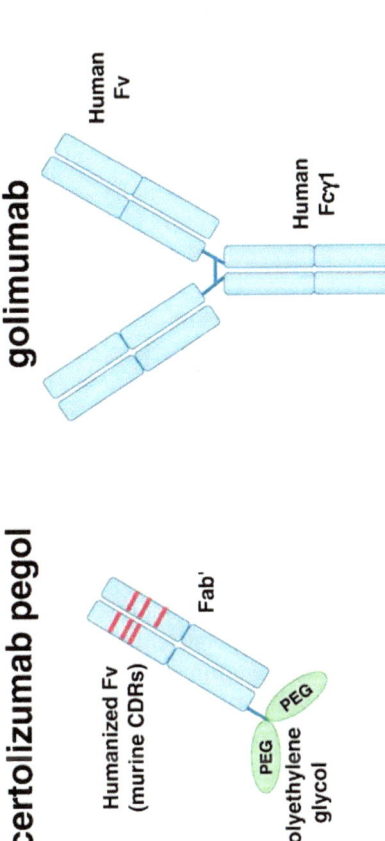

Fig. 7.2 Anti-TNF-α biologic drugs

quality of life and exacerbation rate [13]. In subjects with moderate asthma, the recombinant human-murine chimaeric anti-TNF-α monoclonal antibody infliximab, administered at a dose of 5 mg/Kg on weeks 0, 2 and 6, decreased circadian PEF oscillations and the related disease exacerbations [14]. In a case series referring to a few cases of severe steroid-dependent asthma, Taillé et al. showed that infliximab improved asthma control in six patients treated with this drug for at least 3 months [15]. Moreover, oral corticosteroids could be stopped in four subjects, and the frequency of exacerbations and hospitalizations was remarkably decreased, especially in three patients with brittle asthma. However, two subjects experienced severe adverse effects such as bacterial pneumonia and extension of spreading melanoma [15].

With regard to the use of anti-TNF-α drugs for asthma treatment, a very important study was performed by Wenzel et al. in 309 patients with uncontrolled severe asthma [16]. These authors evaluated the effects of golimumab, a fully human TNF-α blocking antibody, administered at doses of 50, 100 or 200 mg every 4 weeks for 52 weeks. When compared to placebo, golimumab did not elicit any significant improvement in lung function and disease exacerbations. Moreover, serious adverse infectious and neoplastic events were reported, including active tuberculosis, pneumonia, sepsis and several different malignancies such as breast cancer, B-cell lymphoma, metastatic melanoma, cervical carcinoma, renal cell carcinoma, basal cell carcinoma and colon cancer. Therefore, the trial was interrupted, and at present it appears to be very unlikely that anti-TNF-α antibodies will be soon further evaluated for the treatment of severe asthma. The discordances between the studies investigating infliximab and golimumab might be due to phenotypic differences among the enrolled patients, because it is known that subjects with more severe asthma have a greater susceptibility to infections and other comorbidities, which could be exacerbated by TNF-α blockade at a greater extent than individuals with moderate persistent disease. However, a subgroup analysis of the patients enrolled in the golimumab trial demonstrated that the drug was beneficial in older subjects with late-onset asthma and a history of hospitalizations or emergency hospital visits during the year before screening, who also had lower baseline FEV_1 values and a post-bronchodilator FEV_1 increase of >12 % [16]. These observations suggest that patient stratification, based on both clinical and functional parameters, is important in order to identify those patients who could potentially be more responsive to anti-TNF-α therapeutic strategies.

References

1. Brightling C, Berry M, Amrani Y. Targeting TNF-α: a novel therapeutic approach for asthma. J Allergy Clin Immunol. 2008;121:5–10.
2. Lukacs NW, Strieter RM, Chensue SW, et al. TNF-α mediates recruitment of neutrophils and eosinophils during airway inflammation. J Immunol. 1995;154:S411–7.
3. Thomas PS, Yates DH, Barnes PJ. Tumor necrosis factor-α increases airway responsiveness and sputum neutrophilia in normal human subjects. Am J Respir Crit Care Med. 1995;152:76–80.

4. Amrani Y, Panettieri Jr RA, Frossard N, Bronner C. Activation of the TNF-α p55 receptor induces myocyte proliferation and modulates agonist-evoked calcium transients in cultured human tracheal smooth muscle cells. Am J Respir Cell Mol Biol. 1996;15:55–63.

5. Desmouliere A, Geinoz A, Gabbiani F, Gabbiani G. TGF-β1 induces α-smooth muscle actin expression in granulation tissue myofibroblasts and in quiescent and growing cultured fibroblasts. J Cell Biol. 1993;122:103–11.

6. Sullivan DE, Ferris M, Pociask D, Brody AR. Tumor necrosis factor-α induces transforming growth factor-β1 expression in lung fibroblasts through the extracellular signal-regulated kinase pathway. Am J Respir Cell Mol Biol. 2005;32:342–9.

7. Berry MA, Hargadon B, Shelley M, et al. Evidence of a role of tumor necrosis factor-α in refractory asthma. N Engl J Med. 2006;354:697–708.

8. Catal F, Mete E, Tayman C, et al. A human monoclonal anti-TNF alpha antibody reduces airway inflammation and ameliorates lung histology in a murine model of acute asthma. Allergol Immunopathol. 2015;43:14–8.

9. Pelaia G, Vatrella A, Maselli R. The potential of biologics for the treatment of asthma. Nat Rev Drug Discov. 2012;11:958–72.

10. Gallelli L, Busceti MT, Vatrella A, et al. Update on anticytokine treatment for asthma. Biomed Res Int. 2013;2013:104315.

11. Chung KF. Targeting the interleukin pathway in the treatment of asthma. Lancet. 2015;386:1086–96.

12. Howarth PH, Babu KS, Arshad HS, et al. Tumour necrosis factor-α (TNF-α) as a novel therapeutic target in symptomatic corticosteroid dependent asthma. Thorax. 2005;60:1012–8.

13. Holgate ST, Noonan M, Chanez P, et al. Efficacy and safety of etanercept in moderate-to-severe asthma: a randomised, controlled trial. Eur Respir J. 2011;37:1352–9.

14. Erin EM, Leaker BR, Nicholson GC, et al. The effects of a monoclonal antibody directed against tumor necrosis factor-α in asthma. Am J Respir Crit Care Med. 2006;174:753–62.

15. Taillé C, Poulet C, Marchand-Adam S, et al. Monoclonal anti-TNF-α antibodies for severe steroid-dependent asthma: a case series. Open Respir Med J. 2013;7:21–5.

16. Wenzel SE, Barnes PJ, Bleecker ER, et al. A randomized, double-blind, placebo-controlled study of tumor necrosis factor-α blockade in severe persistent asthma. Am J Respir Crit Care Med. 2009;179:549–58.

Biologic Treatments Targeted to Innate Cytokines

8

Interleukin-25 (IL-25), interleukin-33 (IL-33) and thymic stromal lymphopoietin (TSLP) are innate cytokines produced by the airway epithelium, which play a key role in asthma pathobiology by contributing to the development of Th2-mediated adaptive immune responses [1]. In addition to stimulating Th2 cell-dependent allergic bronchial inflammation, IL-25, IL-33 and TSLP are also crucially involved in non-allergic eosinophilic asthma because of their ability to induce type 2 innate lymphoid cells (ILC2s) to produce T2-type cytokines such as IL-5, IL-9 and IL-13 [2]. Therefore, IL-25, IL-33 and TSLP are suitable targets for antiasthma biological therapies [3].

Anti-IL-25 Monoclonal Antibodies

IL-25, also known as IL-17E, is a member of the IL-17 cytokine family which induces eosinophilic inflammation by stimulating the production of IL-5 and eotaxin [4, 5]. High plasma levels of IL-25 are detectable in allergic asthmatic patients, whose eosinophils are characterized by an increased expression of the IL-25 receptor [6]. In a mouse model of allergic asthma, an anti-IL-25 monoclonal antibody prevented airway hyperresponsiveness and significantly decreased IL-5 and IL-13 production, airway eosinophil infiltration, goblet cell hyperplasia and serum IgE levels [7]. However, this experimental therapeutic approach has not yet been extended to asthmatic patients.

Anti-IL-33 Therapies

IL-33 is an IL-1-like pro-inflammatory cytokine which promotes the production of IL-4, IL-5 and IL-13 [8–10]. IL-33 is up-regulated in patients with severe asthma and exerts its biological effects via activation of its own ST2 receptor [11, 12]. In mice, anti-IL-33 monoclonal antibodies have been shown to attenuate allergen-induced eosinophilic airway inflammation, mucus hypersecretion and production of Th2 cytokines [13]. Furthermore, allergic inflammation and airway hyperresponsiveness can be inhibited in mice by antibodies directed towards the ST2 receptor [14]. However, the potential antiasthmatic effects arising from the blockade of either IL-33 or its ST2 receptor should be carefully balanced against the eventual

© Springer International Publishing Switzerland 2017
G. Pelaia et al., *Asthma: Targeted Biological Therapies*,
DOI 10.1007/978-3-319-46007-9_8

risks due to suppression of the physiological benefits mediated by this cytokine, including wound healing, antiviral immunity and possibly protection against cardio-vascular diseases [12].

Anti-TSLP Treatments

Another pro-inflammatory mediator released from airway epithelial cells is TSLP, an IL-7-related cytokine which stimulates dendritic cells to produce chemokines that recruit and activate Th2 lymphocytes [15]. In asthmatic subjects, the airway epithelium is characterized by an increased expression of TSLP, which induces bronchial and blood eosinophilia via stimulation of IL-5 and IL-13 production [16, 17]. In addition to contributing to the development of eosinophilic airway inflam-mation, TSLP is also involved in viral-induced lung inflammation and fibroblast-dependent bronchial remodelling [18, 19].

In a mouse model of allergic asthma, intratracheal administration of an antibody targeting the TSLP receptor, performed before allergen challenge, significantly reduced eosinophilic airway inflammation, goblet cell hyperplasia and production of Th2 cytokines; these effects were mediated by inhibition of maturation and migration of airway dendritic cells, which were not able anymore to drive Th2-dependent cellular responses [20]. More interestingly, a fully human anti-TSLP monoclonal antibody (AMG-157) was recently evaluated in a double-blind study carried out in 31 patients with mild allergic asthma, who were randomly assigned to receive either placebo or three intravenous monthly doses (700 mg) of AMG-157 [21]. FEV_1 decreases during late asthmatic responses induced by allergen challenge were 34.0 % and 45.9 % smaller on day 42 and day 84, respectively, when recorded in the AMG-157 group in comparison to the placebo arm. Moreover, AMG-157 significantly reduced blood and sputum eosinophil counts, as well as fractional exhaled nitric oxide levels [21].

References

1. Pelaia G, Vatrella A, Busceti MT, et al. Cellular mechanisms underlying eosinophilic and neu-trophilic airway inflammation in asthma. Mediators Inflamm. 2015;2015:879783.
2. Holgate ST, Wenzel S, Postma DS, et al. Asthma. Nat Rev Dis Primers. 2015;1:15025.
3. Mitchell PD, El-Gammal A, O'Byrne PM. Emerging monoclonal antibodies as targeted inno-vative therapeutic approaches to asthma. Clin Pharmacol Ther. 2016;99:38–48.
4. Tamachi T, Maezawa Y, Ikeda K, et al. Interleukin 25 in allergic airway inflammation. Int Arch Allergy Immunol. 2006;140 Suppl 1:59–62.
5. Cheng D, Xue Z, Yi L, et al. Interleukin 25 is a key mediator in Th2-high, corticosteroid-responsive asthma. Am Allergy Immunol. 2006;140:59–62.
6. Tang W, Smith SG, Beaudin S, et al. IL-25 and IL-25 receptor expression on eosinophils from subjects with allergic asthma. Int Arch Allergy Immunol. 2014;163:5–10.
7. Ballantyne SJ, Barlow JL, Jolin HE, et al. Blocking IL-25 prevents airway hyperresponsive-ness in allergic asthma. J Allergy Clin Immunol. 2007;120:1324–31.

8. Haraldsen G, Balogh J, Pollheimer J, et al. Interleukin-33 – cytokine of dual function or novel alarmin? Trends Immunol. 2009;30:227–33.

9. Yagami A, Orihara K, Morita H, et al. IL-33 mediates inflammatory responses in human lung tissue cells. J Immunol. 2010;185:5743–50.

10. Nabe T. Interleukin(IL)-33: new therapeutic target for atopic diseases. J Pharmacol Sci. 2014;126:85–91.

11. Prefontaine D, Lajoie-Kadoch S, Foley S, et al. Increased expression of IL-33 in severe asthma: evidence of expression by airway smooth muscle cells. J Immunol. 2009;183:5094–103.

12. Hardman C, Ogg G. Interleukin-33, friend and foe in type-2 immune responses. Curr Opin Immunol. 2016;42:16–24.

13. Mizutani N, Nabe T, Yoshino S. Interleukin-33 and alveolar macrophages contribute to the mechanisms underlying the exacerbation of IgE-mediated airway inflammation and remodelling in mice. Immunology. 2013;139:205–18.

14. Kearley J, Buckland KF, Mathie SA, Lloyd CM. Resolution of allergic inflammation and airway hyperreactivity is dependent upon disruption of the T1/ST2-IL-33 pathway. Am J Respir Crit Care Med. 2009;179:772–81.

15. Liu YJ, Soumelis V, Watanabe N, et al. TSLP: an epithelial cell cytokine that regulates T cell differentiation by conditioning dendritic cell maturation. Annu Rev Immunol. 2007;25:193–219.

16. Ying S, O'Connor B, Ratoff J, et al. Expression and cellular provenance of thymic stromal lymphopoietin and chemokines in patients with severe asthma and chronic obstructive pulmonary disease. J Immunol. 2008;181:2790–8.

17. Zhou B, Comeau MR, De Smedt T, et al. Thymic stromal lymphopoietin as a key initiator of allergic airway inflammation in mice. Nat Immunol. 2005;6:1047–53.

18. Lay MK, Comeau MR, De Smedt T, et al. Human metapneumovirus infection activates the TSLP pathway which drives excessive pulmonary inflammation and viral replication in mice. Eur J Immunol. 2015;45:1680–95.

19. Wu J, Liu F, Zhao J, et al. Thymic stromal lymphopoietin promotes asthmatic airway remodelling in human lung fibroblast cells through STAT3 signalling pathway. Cell Biochem Funct. 2013;31:496–503.

20. Shi L, Leu SW, Xu F, et al. Local blockade of TSLP receptor alleviated allergic disease by regulating airway dendritic cells. Clin Immunol. 2008;129:202–10.

21. Gauvreau GM, O'Byrne PM, Boulet LP, et al. Effects of an anti-TSLP antibody on allergen-induced asthmatic responses. N Engl J Med. 2014;370:2102–10.

Potentially suitable targets for antiasthma treatments also include other pro-inflammatory cytokines such as interleukin-9 (IL-9), granulocyte-macrophage colony-stimulating factor (GM-CSF) as well as interleukin-17 (IL-17) and interleukin-23 (IL-23) [1–4].

Anti-IL-9 Monoclonal Antibodies

IL-9 is a pleiotropic Th2 cytokine overexpressed in asthmatic airways, where it exerts its biological actions on Th2 lymphocytes, B cells, mast cells, eosinophils and airway epithelial cells [5]. In particular, IL-9 induces mast cell proliferation and mucus hyperplasia [6]. In allergen-sensitized mice, anti-IL-9 antibodies attenuated airway inflammation by decreasing the numbers of mast cells and eosinophils, inhibited bronchial hyperresponsiveness to methacholine and reduced airway remodelling by downregulating the expression of profibrotic agents such as transforming growth factor-$\beta 1$ (TGF-$\beta 1$), fibroblast growth factor-2 (FGF-2) and vascular endothelial growth factor (VEGF) [7, 8]. In healthy subjects, the humanized anti-IL-9 antibody MEDI-528 was safe and well tolerated, being characterized by linear pharmacokinetics when administered either intravenously or subcutaneously [9]. In one of two randomized phase 2a studies conducted in patients with mild-to-moderate asthma, MEDI-528 induced a trend towards an improvement in Asthma Quality of Life Questionnaire (AQLQ) scores and a decrease in asthma exacerbation rates [10]. The second of these two clinical trials showed that 50 mg of MEDI-528, given subcutaneously twice weekly, exerted a protective effect against exercise-induced bronchoconstriction [10]. However, a more recent placebo-controlled study carried out in 327 asthmatic patients demonstrated that MEDI-528, administered subcutaneously as add on-therapy at dosages of either 30, 100 or 300 mg twice weekly for 4 weeks, did not significantly change Asthma Control Questionnaire 6 (ACQ-6) scores, respiratory function and asthma exacerbation rates [11]. Therefore, the potential antiasthma effects of IL-9 blockade need to be further evaluated.

© Springer International Publishing Switzerland 2017
G. Pelaia et al., *Asthma: Targeted Biological Therapies*,
DOI 10.1007/978-3-319-46007-9_9

Anti-GM-CSF Drugs

GM-CSF plays a key role in eosinophil differentiation and survival and is overexpressed in asthmatic airways [6]. In a mouse model of allergic asthma, intranasal administration of an anti-GM-CSF polyclonal antibody significantly dampened airway inflammation, mucus production and bronchial hyperresponsiveness [12]. Furthermore, a human anti-GM-CSF monoclonal IgG1 antibody (MT203) reduced the survival and activation of peripheral human eosinophils [13]. Recently, the effects on lung function of an anti-GM-CSF monoclonal antibody (KB003) were evaluated in adult asthmatics inadequately controlled by inhaled/oral corticosteroids and long-acting β_2-adrenergic agonists, who received seven intravenous infusions of either placebo or KB003 (400 mg) at baseline and at weeks 2, 4, 8, 12, 16 and 20, respectively [14]. Overall, KB003 did not significantly change FEV_1 values at week 24. However, at several different time points, anti-GM-CSF therapy induced significant FEV_1 increases in some patient subgroups including subjects with blood eosinophil counts ≥ 300 cells/μl, or post-bronchodilator FEV_1 reversibility $\geq 20\%$ or baseline $FEV_1 \leq 50\%$ of predicted values [14].

Anti-IL-17 and Anti-IL-23 Therapies

IL-17A and IL-17 F are pro-inflammatory cytokines produced by Th17 lymphocytes; they play a central role in neutrophilic inflammation, and their expression levels in bronchial biopsies correlate with asthma severity, especially in patients with neutrophilic corticosteroid-resistant disease [15, 16]. In particular, IL-17A and IL-17 F induce airway epithelial cells and subepithelial fibroblasts to release powerful neutrophil chemoattractants such as CXCL8 and CXCL1 [3]. In a mouse model of allergic asthma, anti-IL-17 monoclonal antibodies were able to significantly lower the numbers of neutrophils, eosinophils and lymphocytes in bronchoalveolar lavage fluid (BALF) [17].

In a randomized, placebo-controlled study involving 302 patients with severe asthma, inadequately controlled by inhaled corticosteroids and long-acting β_2-adrenergic agonists, the fully human monoclonal antibody brodalumab, targeted against the IL-17 receptor A, was tested at different subcutaneous dosages (140, 210 and 280 mg), administered every 2 weeks for 10 weeks [18]. Brodalumab did not improve asthma symptoms and FEV_1. However, in a subpopulation of subjects with a high reversibility documented by a post-bronchodilator FEV_1 increase of 20% or more, a significant improvement in ACQ score was detected at the 210 mg, but not at the 280 mg dosage. Anyway, a subsequent phase 2b trial enrolling patients with this asthma phenotype was interrupted because of a lack of evident benefits [3]. The human anti-IL-17A monoclonal antibody secukinumab is currently under investigation in patients with uncontrolled asthma [4]. An alternative biologic strategy targets the IL-17-regulating cytokine IL-23, which can be neutralized by a monoclonal antibody capable of inhibiting antigen-dependent recruitment of neutrophils, eosinophils and lymphocytes into the airways of sensitized mice [19]. In this animal model of asthma, a further therapeutic approach is based on RNA interference-mediated knockdown of IL-23, which significantly reduced BALF numbers of both neutrophils and eosinophils [20]. However, extreme caution should be paid to the experimental blockade of the IL-23/IL-17 axis, which is also implicated in immune protection against infectious and carcinogenic agents [21]. Therefore, inactivation of this cytokine pathway could expose to an enhanced risk of developing opportunistic infections and cancer.

References

1. Pelaia G, Vatrella A, Maselli R. The potential of biologics for the treatment of asthma. Nat Rev Drug Discov. 2012;11:958–72.
2. Gallelli L, Busceti MT, Vatrella A, et al. Update on anticytokine treatment for asthma. Biomed Res Int. 2013;2013:104315.
3. Chung KF. Targeting the interleukin pathway in the treatment of asthma. Lancet. 2015;386:1086–96.
4. Mitchell PD, El-Gammal A, O'Byrne PM. Emerging monoclonal antibodies as targeted innovative therapeutic approaches to asthma. Clin Pharmacol Ther. 2016;99:38–48.
5. Xing J, Wu Y, Ni B. Th9: a new player in asthma pathogenesis? J Asthma. 2011;48:115–25.
6. Barnes PJ. The cytokine network in asthma and chronic obstructive pulmonary disease. J Clin Invest. 2008;118:3546–56.
7. Cheng G, Arima M, Honda K, et al. Anti-interleukin-9 antibody treatment inhibits airway inflammation and hyperreactivity in mouse asthma model. Am J Respir Crit Care Med. 2002;166:409–16.
8. Kearley J, Eriefalt JS, Andersson C, et al. IL-9 governs allergen-induced mast cell numbers in the lung and chronic remodelling of the airways. Am J Respir Crit Care Med. 2011;183:865–75.
9. White B, Leon F, White W, Robbie G. Two first-in-human, open-label, phase I dose-escalation safety trials of MEDI-528, a monoclonal antibody against interleukin-9 in healthy volunteers. Clin Ther. 2009;31:728–40.
10. Parker JM, Oh CK, LaForce C, et al. Safety profile and clinical activity of multiple subcutaneous doses of MEDI-528, a humanized anti-interleukin-9 monoclonal antibody, in two randomized phase 2a studies in subjects with asthma. BMC Pulm Med. 2011;11:14.
11. Oh CK, Leigh R, McLaurin KK, et al. A randomized, controlled trial to evaluate the effect of an anti-interleukin-9 monoclonal antibody in adults with uncontrolled asthma. Respir Res. 2013;14:93.
12. Yamashita N, Tashimo H, Ishida H, et al. Attenuation of airway hyperresponsiveness in a murine asthma model by neutralization of granulocyte-macrophage colony-stimulating factor (GM-CSF). Cell Immunol. 2002;219:92–7.
13. Krinner EM, Raum T, Petsch S, et al. A human monoclonal IgG1 potently neutralizing the pro-inflammatory cytokine GM-CSF. Mol Immunol. 2007;44:916–25.
14. Molfino NA, Kuna P, Leff JA, et al. Phase 2, randomised placebo-controlled trial to evaluate the efficacy and safety of an anti-GM-CSF antibody (KB003) in patients with inadequately controlled asthma. BMJ Open. 2016;6:e007709.
15. Al Ramly W, Prefontaine D, Chouiali F, et al. T(H)17-associated cytokines (IL-17A and IL-17F) in severe asthma. J Allergy Clin Immunol. 2009;123:1185–7.
16. Vazquez-Tello A, Halwani R, Hamid Q, Al-Muhsen S. Glucocorticoid receptor-b up-regulation and steroid resistance induction by IL-17 and IL-23 cytokine stimulation in peripheral mononuclear cells. J Clin Immunol. 2013;33:466–78.

17. Hellings PW, Kasran A, Liu Z, et al. Interleukin-17 orchestrates the granulocyte influx into airways after allergen inhalation in a mouse model of allergic asthma. Am J Respir Cell Mol Biol. 2003;28:42–50.
18. Busse WW, Holgate S, Kerwin E, et al. Randomized, double-blind, placebo-controlled study of brodalumab, a human anti-IL-17 receptor monoclonal antibody, in moderate to severe asthma. Am J Respir Crit Care Med. 2013;188:1294–302.
19. Wakashin H, Hirose K, Maezawa Y, et al. IL-23 and Th17 cells enhance Th2-cell-mediated eosinophilic airway inflammation in mice. Am J Respir Crit Care Med. 2008;178:1023–32.
20. Li Y, Sun M, Cheng H, et al. Silencing IL-23 expression by a small hairpin RNA protects against asthma in mice. Exp Mol Med. 2011;43:197–204.
21. Park SJ, Lee YC. Interleukin-17 regulation: an attractive therapeutic approach for asthma. Respir Res. 2010;11:78.

Conclusions and Future Perspectives

During the last years, asthma treatment has entered a new fascinating era of trust-worthy realities and promising perspectives [1]. These significant advances have been made possible by the recent relevant progress achieved towards a better understanding of the cellular and molecular mechanisms underlying asthma pathobiology [2, 3]. Undoubtedly, the most important new therapeutic tools available for the treatment of asthma, especially with regard to the more severe disease phenotypes, are biologic drugs [4]. Indeed, omalizumab and mepolizumab are already included in the step 5 of GINA guidelines for asthma management [5], and reslizumab has been recently approved by FDA [6]. Moreover, the current intense development of molecular-targeted therapies, many of which are undergoing advanced stages of clinical investigation, will probably lead in the next future to the introduction in real life of several other biologics indicated for asthma treatment [7–11].

Of course, an accurate phenotypic stratification is absolutely required for implementation of antiasthma biological therapies. Indeed, differently from corticosteroids that interfere with multiple pro-inflammatory pathways widely involved in asthma pathophysiology, biologics usually neutralize specific pathogenic targets, which are relevant for a given phenotype/endotype. For example, atopic patients who are not adequately controlled by corticosteroids can greatly benefit from anti-IgE treatment with omalizumab. Either allergic or non-allergic subjects with eosinophilic, corticosteroid-resistant asthma may experience significant clinical improvements by receiving biologic therapies targeting IL-5 or its receptor. High blood levels of periostin can help to select asthmatic patients potentially responsive to the therapeutic effects of anti-IL-13 monoclonal antibodies. Moreover, very promising appear to be the perspective approaches aimed to inhibit the effects of the innate cytokines IL-25, IL-33 and TSLP, which are very important in the initial priming of T2-type airway inflammation; such cytokine-based biologic strategies could thus make it possible to disrupt the crosstalk between innate and adaptive immune responses, which in susceptible individuals contributes to the development of severe and difficult-to-treat subtypes of asthma.

In this regard, it is essential to utilize reliable biomarkers, easily measurable in daily clinical practice, which can provide a useful help to characterize specific asthma phenotypes/endotypes and predict their responses to biological treatments [12, 13]. Indeed, this approach allows to outline, across the heterogeneity of asthma pathophysiology, the clinical and biological profiles that make up the individual expressions of this disease, as well as the possible success of personalized therapies,

© Springer International Publishing Switzerland 2017
G. Pelaia et al., *Asthma: Targeted Biological Therapies*,
DOI 10.1007/978-3-319-46007-9_10

thus hopefully satisfying the unmet medical needs of patients with difficult-to-control asthma. Within this context, biologic drugs can play a relevant role by providing a diversified choice of tailored antiasthma medications. During the last few years, basic and clinical research strategies have identified many attractive molecular targets for asthma treatment. In particular, IgE- and cytokine-targeted therapies, added to conventional treatments and used according to the patient's individual requirements, could lead to considerable improvements in the control of severe asthma.

Unfortunately, the most common available biomarkers, such as IgE, blood/sputum eosinophils, FeNO and periostin, only characterize the so-called 'Th2-high' or 'type 2' subtypes of airway inflammation, mainly referring to eosinophilic asthma [14]. Hence, with the debatable exception of sputum neutrophilia, there has been much less success in identifying biomarkers potentially useful to delineate 'Th2-low' or 'non-Th2'/'non-type 2' asthma. The lack of reliable biomarkers for non-type 2 asthma has considerably delayed the development of effective therapeutic strategies targeted to this phenotypic/endotypic disease pattern. Moreover, because of possible molecular interactions between Th2 and non-Th2 mechanisms [9], also the mixed eosinophilic/neutrophilic profiles of severe asthma deserve attention in order to develop two-sided approaches. Another challenge refers to the detection of eventually useful biomarkers in order to predict the therapeutic response to biological treatments in terms of inhibition of airway remodelling. In this regard, it is noteworthy to point out that galectin-3 has been recognized as a potential predictor of omalizumab effectiveness in reducing the thickness of bronchial wall in atopic patients with severe asthma [15].

Finally, because it is frequently reported that the blockade of a single cytokine or mediator can result in only partial efficacy, a further research perspective might explore, in carefully selected asthmatic patients, the effects of different cocktails of biologics targeting several different pathogenic pathways underlying complex asthma phenotypes [7]. Anyway, there is no doubt that in the coming decades biologic drugs will represent a key cornerstone in the management of severe asthma.

References

1. Charriot J, Vachier I, Halimi L, et al. Future treatments for asthma. Eur Respir J. 2016;25:77–92.
2. Holgate ST, Wenzel S, Postma DS, et al. Asthma. Nat Rev Dis Primers. 2015;1:15025.
3. Pelaia G, Vatrella A, Busceti MT, et al. Cellular mechanisms underlying eosinophilic and neutrophilic airway inflammation in asthma. Mediators Inflamm. 2015;2015:879783.
4. Ray A, Raundhal M, Oriss TB, et al. Current concepts of severe asthma. J Clin Invest. 2016;126:2394–403.
5. Global strategy for asthma management and prevention. Global Initiative for Asthma (GINA). 2016. Available from: http://www.ginasthma.org/.
6. Pelaia G, Vatrella A, Busceti MT, et al. Role of biologics in severe eosinophilic asthma – focus on reslizumab. Ther Clin Risk Manag. 2016;12:1075–82.
7. Pelaia G, Vatrella A, Maselli R. The potential of biologics for the treatment of asthma. Nat Rev Drug Discov. 2012;11:958–72.

8. Gallelli L, Busceti MT, Vatrella A, et al. Update on anticytokine treatment for asthma. Biomed Res Int. 2013;2013:104315.

9. Chung KF. Targeting the interleukin pathway in the treatment of asthma. Lancet. 2015;386:1086–96.

10. Heck S, Nguyen J, Le DD, et al. Pharmacological therapy of bronchial asthma: the role of biologicals. Int Arch Allergy Immunol. 2015;168:241–52.

11. Mitchell PD, El-Gammal A, O'Byrne PM. Emerging monoclonal antibodies as targeted innovative therapeutic approaches to asthma. Clin Pharmacol Ther. 2016;99:38–48.

12. Szefler SJ, Wenzel S, Brown R. Asthma outcomes: biomarkers. J Allergy Clin Immunol. 2012;129(3 Suppl):S9–S23.

13. Staton TL, Choy DF, Arron JR. Biomarkers in the clinical development of asthma therapies. Biomark Med. 2016;10:165–76.

14. Wenzel SE. Emergence of biomolecular pathways to define novel asthma phenotypes. Type-2 immunity and beyond. Am J Respir Cell Mol Biol. 2016;55:1–4.

15. Mauri P, Riccio AM, Rossi R, et al. Proteomics of bronchial biopsies: galectin-3 as a predictive biomarker of airway remodelling modulation in omalizumab-treated severe asthma patients. Immunol Lett. 2014;162:2–10.